THE GOO

Nilesha Chauvet is a British Indian novelist and short-story writer. She is also the managing director of GOOD, which advises commercial brands on purpose and helps charities to raise millions of pounds for good causes. A graduate of Faber Academy, Nilesha also studied creative writing at Curtis Brown Creative and City Lit. She read philosophy and theology at Oxford and is an ordained interfaith minister. Her debut novel, *Her Two Lives*, was awarded a prestigious London Writers Award and was shortlisted for the Spotlight First Novel Award and the McDermid Debut Award.

*by the same author*

HER TWO LIVES

NILESHA CHAUVET

# THE GOOD PATIENT

faber

First published in the UK in 2026
by Faber & Faber Ltd
The Bindery, 51 Hatton Garden
London EC1N 8HN

Typeset by Faber & Faber Ltd
Printed and bound by CPI Group (UK) Ltd, Croydon CR0 4YY

All rights reserved
© Nilesha Chauvet, 2025

The right of Nilesha Chauvet to be identified as author of this work has been asserted in accordance with Section 77 of the Copyright, Designs and Patents Act 1988

*This is a work of fiction. All of the characters, organisations and events portrayed in this novel are either products of the author's imagination or are used fictitiously*

A CIP record for this book
is available from the British Library

ISBN 978-0-571-38217-0

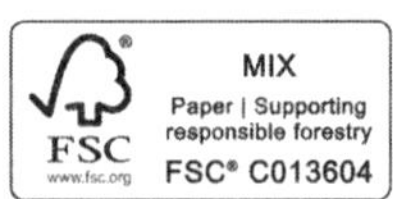


Printed and bound in the UK on FSC® certified paper in line with our continuing commitment to ethical business practices, sustainability and the environment.
**For further information see faber.co.uk/environmental-policy**

Our authorised representative in the EU for product safety is
Easy Access System Europe, Mustamäe tee 50, 10621 Tallinn, Estonia
gpsr.requests@easproject.com

2 4 6 8 10 9 7 5 3 1

'The very first requirement in a hospital is that it should do the sick no harm.'

Florence Nightingale

*For nurses, everywhere.*

# PROLOGUE

Barrister James Lockwood, closing speech for the prosecution. Wednesday July 19th, 2023. 15.00 hrs.

*If you want to get away with murder, kill someone expected to die. If you want to escape guilt-free, kill someone people despise.*

*Members of the jury, over the past seven weeks the defence has led you to believe that this trial is about a nurse whose primary motivation lay in caring for her patients. That one terrible night, Nina Dabral found herself pushed to the edge, mistreated, unsupported, suffering post-pandemic stress. No longer was she able to discern right from wrong, she says.*

*But I urge you to consider the evidence. To park to one side the stories you may have heard about the tragic demise of our healthcare system. The significant toll this is taking on otherwise good nurses. Consider the facts. Consider what she did that night with her own hands when she could, so easily, have chosen differently.*

*This trial is about a woman who deliberately failed a promising young man. A man whom she despised and misjudged, who might otherwise be alive had it not been for her actions. That night, her primary motivation was murder. That, ladies and gentlemen, is what this trial is about.*

Seated in the dock at the Old Bailey, it's difficult to take it all in. I've waited six months for this moment to arrive, but I still feel hopelessly defeated. They remanded me into custody, made me live under the regime of the guilty. I tell you, I can't go back, I really can't. But I fear their minds are decided.

It's easy to try a key worker in the court of public opinion. Alarmist headlines guiding head and heart in place of empathy and kindness. I'm an angel of death to some. A casualty of the National *Hell* Service to others. A good nurse gone bad who simply cracked under the pressure. What fascinates yet horrifies people in equal measure is how my actions could escalate from neglect to bloody murder.

I glance down at my hands. My wrists chafe and burn from where the handcuffs cut into my skin. I close my eyes, trembling from the endless hours of cross-examination. The judge sits opposite, her gown crumpled, face crimson.

'Nina Dabral . . .' She eases herself gently forward. 'I must tell you that the charges of which you are accused are extremely serious. Have you any final words you'd like to say before the jury is left to consider its final verdict?'

I bite my lip and taste blood. I know that no matter what I say, the administration of justice is not about truth anymore. It's about who the judge or jury likes. The information they *selectively* believe.

'Nothing, your honour,' I croak, growing convinced that they're in on it too, this determination to have me silenced.

I cross my heart and inwardly swear that one day, I'll tell the world my version.

# 1

My feet dragged as I walked up the concrete steps of Newgate Hospital. I reminded myself that being here made a difference. I worked thirty-seven and a half hours each week, every minute accounted for, every second supposedly meaningful.

It was an October evening. The nation mourned the passing of Queen Elizabeth II. The announcement of a new prime minister after the last one proved a disaster. The hospital smelled of chlorine, bleach, and disinfectant, where in their enthusiasm for the coming Diwali celebrations, the cleaners had been heavy-handed.

I walked through the main reception, past the closed gift shop streaming with balloons, ribbons, and colourful get-well cards. Past the disabled toilet where patients had been known to inject heroin in cubicles, others having sex with strangers. I turned right, moving through the corridor that ran like an artery through the main body of the hospital, questioning how much more of this I could take. I did the only thing I thought might help. I repeated my daily affirmation:

*I am kind and loving to myself. I am conscious of how I feel. I am energised and ready, no matter how difficult things appear. I exist only to do good, to help heal my sick patients.*

I stepped into the lift, pressing the button for the second floor. Filmed in sweat, my face prickled as it met the air-conditioned cold.

Inside Florence Nightingale ASU, Reggie, a jaunty cleaner, was mopping the grey vinyl floors.

'Nina! Ready for another busy night?'

'Born ready,' I said. I nodded to the floor: wet and streaky. 'You're doing a great job there.'

'You know me.' Reggie smiled coyly. He removed a pencil snuck behind his ear, placing it in his breast pocket. 'No matter what shit goes on in here, I leave things *sweet* like poetry.'

In the distance, that familiar, almost comforting sound of patients – coughs, the crinkle of plastic mattresses. The beep-beep-beep of heart monitors, another reminder of how important my work was. Then, unmistakably, the sound of a woman crying.

I hurried into the side room next to the staff kitchen amid the low hum of white noise, the steady thrum of trolleys rolling.

Preeti was seated on a sofa in the far-right corner. She peered into her phone. Sandra, a senior nurse, had a cold compress pressed to her eye. I jolted, a moment of blank, trying to take in what had happened. 'Are you hurt?'

She rose, shakily, walking towards the mirror. Peering at her face, she lowered her hand to reveal an angry swelling.

'It's nothing,' she said.

'It doesn't look like nothing!'

'A patient punched her as she tried to take blood,' Preeti cut in. 'Sandra did nothing wrong. She was just doing her job!'

My chest grew tight as I thought, *It's starting*. The blood of gang violence from the streets was now seeping into the supposedly safe space of the hospital. I reminded myself to keep calm. The last thing I needed was to alarm the others. No good would come from blaming the police stationed in A&E for not doing enough – though that was precisely how I saw it.

'We need to report whoever did this,' I said, painfully aware that my shift had barely begun, yet here I was, now having to deal with an assault against one of my nurses. 'Have you called Barry?'

'Not yet,' said Preeti, hauling herself up.

'Why not? What good is having the police here if they don't *do* anything? It's bad enough that they can't deal with what's going on *outside* in Levinstone, let alone *inside* this hospital.'

DC Barry Coombs was referred to by many as the town's black Elvis. Less to do with his deep voice, more to do with his sideburns, black boots, and annoyingly noisy buckles.

'Vivian Butler. Bed five. Brought in with a knife wound,' said Preeti. 'Look . . .' She clambered towards me. 'She's on Instagram. Nasty piece of work. Linked to that gang. Probably responsible for that TikTok video that went viral.'

I grabbed the phone, unable to stop myself scrolling through the pictures. I saw a woman no older than eighteen, dolled up, pouting in a hoodie. She wore a red bandana; pink lips, full and glossy.

I handed the phone back. 'Put it away,' I mumbled. 'It's distracting when there's so much going on.'

'Stone Killaz. It's what they call themselves, isn't it?' Preeti's voice trailed as I moved closer to Sandra.

'Let's get you cleaned up. If you'd prefer to go home, that's fine. But we need to follow procedure.'

*Procedure. Endless bloody procedure.*

'I'll log the incident and report it to the police. I'll also let Barbara know that we need to review safety as an immediate action.'

Sandra nodded.

'All Sandra wanted to do was another blood test, and Vivian was like "Why do I have to do another one? I've already done three in triage!" Then she completely lost it.' Preeti slipped her phone into her pocket.

I inspected Sandra's cheek, the side swollen, her swan-like neck pink and rashy. 'There's bruising but no serious damage,' I said. 'You'll have one hell of a shiner, though.'

Sandra pulled away. 'It's fine. Anong's called in sick. Best if I stay here.'

Reluctantly, I agreed. The last thing I needed was to be a nurse down.

I asked Preeti to assist Sandra – assuming she could tear herself away from her phone. I left the two of them alone to enter the changing room next door.

Wearily, I placed my bag down to catch my breath. Glancing at my scrubs hanging up, freshly laundered the night before, I moved closer. My fingers swept across the fabric, the material thin and flimsy. Hardly adequate protection against a punch, a stab, even a spray of bullets. What kind of job was this where I now feared for my own safety?

But I was a nurse. No matter what, I knew I must keep calm and carry on. So much of my life had been unstable. Here was something solid to hold on to. I felt an overwhelming sense of loyalty tugging at my core. The NHS was part of my identity, just as the hospital was the beating heart of this town.

I changed into my scrubs, pinning my name tag onto my breast.

*No matter how difficult things might appear, I exist only to do good, to help heal my sick patients . . .*

In the corridor, Matron Barbara Dean was talking to Ravi Parmar, a gangly, overly enthusiastic hospital pharmacist. They dashed past me at considerable speed. I waved to catch their attention and they stopped, Barbara checking her pager, an iPad pressed to her chest, Ravi, visibly aggrieved that he hadn't quite finished his sentence.

'Sorry to interrupt,' I said.

Matron nodded for Ravi to leave. Ravi did so, but reluctantly.

Barbara's hair was short, freshly cut and curled. She looked good, a little younger than her fifty-seven years, and yet she wore the expression of someone carrying the heavy weight of the world.

'There's been an incident,' I said. 'I need to make you aware of it.'

Barbara straightened her back. 'Come with me,' she said, nodding in the direction of her office.

Maria Gonzalez, the ward manager, appeared. Consumed in thought, she stared down at her shoes as she walked. I felt wary, knowing how she liked to spring issues on us at the last minute. But thankfully, she carried on past us.

Inside the airless room, once a patient toilet, the walls were painted egg yellow. Barbara placed her iPad on the table and sat down, an arm straying onto her desk next to a pile of papers.

'This time it's Sandra,' I said. 'Punched by a patient angry about her taking blood.'

'Christ. That's two this month. Has the incident been logged?'

'About to do it now.'

Barbara removed her glasses and took the tip of one arm, biting on the end. She stared out into the distance, eyes baggy. 'I'll raise it urgently. Get Barry up here with the managers to review safety procedures.'

I nodded. 'On it.'

'Oh – but best not to talk about it too much,' said Barbara. 'It'll only unsettle the others. Getting even temp nurses through the door is proving difficult.'

She was right, of course. Drawing attention to problems would simply undermine efforts to keep things positive. But she was missing the point. I took a seat on a plastic chair opposite. 'There is one more thing,' I said.

'Oh?' She peered at me.

'I know you know this, but . . . we need more staff.'

Barbara glanced to the side, towards the window. 'It's not like I don't feel your frustration. But we need strong justification for additional spend. New targets have already been set. Only essential cover is possible.'

'But that makes no sense.' My voice quivered. 'We've got an influx of patients who are disorderly and *criminal*. It's only going to get worse.'

Barbara shot me a look. 'Who and what patients are isn't relevant. Here, we treat them equally. If the workload is concerning you, that's a separate issue.' She folded her arms. 'Everyone counts, no matter who they are – good or bad, regardless of their background.'

I swallowed hard. 'I understand.'

I knew my nursing code. I abided by its rules more closely than most.

'Good to hear,' Barbara said.

'All I'm saying is that *I am* thinking about improving the lives of others, working together for patients . . .' I could have gone on, quoting the Code, but I felt my lower lip tremble. 'It's hard putting them first in our current situation.' Barbara knew about the problems we faced, yet refused to address them head-on. 'We should speak to the management. Push for more spend. They must surely see the rise in admissions.'

Barbara shook her head like it might be too painful to listen.

'We're an ASU. Patients should be in and out in seventy-two hours,' I continued. But I knew I was losing ground. Barbara's face said it all.

'Workloads were already reviewed,' she said, 'staffing levels agreed and implemented.'

She placed her glasses on the table. 'You know it's been difficult financially. We're doing what we can in a very difficult situation.'

I felt my face burn, wondering whether this is what happens after twenty-five years in a job. Compliance, lack of challenge, subservience, even.

Barbara pursed her lips. 'As nurse in charge, you'll know our new CEO has set stricter targets. The priority is efficiency, cost control. Ensuring the smooth implementation of suppliers and new processes. To get *his* support, and the support of the managers, you need to talk about new streams of revenue.'

I felt my stomach sink. Richard Lonsdale with his frigging new targets. I hated him.

'It's the kind of thinking needed for an elevation to the next pay band,' Barbara said. 'What Richard wants is to encourage a greater sense of commercial enterprise. It's why he's driven through so many changes.'

There was a knock on the door. Maria didn't wait for an answer before ducking her head round.

'Don't suppose you have a minute?' She looked straight at Barbara, ignoring me. 'It's about the new process for MediCentral.'

'I'm almost done,' said Barbara.

Maria nodded and opened the door wider.

It was hopeless. I left the office to log the incident concerning Vivian and to continue nursing my patients.

In the ward, the air was chilly, as if a window had been left open for too long, the wet-pavement smell from outside mingling with the scent of citrus cleaner.

I settled into work, completing a handover with three nurses I'd never met from Platinum Care.

Newgate's ASU had ten cubicles, twenty acute surgical inpatient beds, two procedure rooms, and a surgical ambulatory clinic where discharged patients were reviewed. But I could hardly remember a time when there were enough nurses. Standing at the nurse's station, I scanned my patient list on the PC screen. So many of them were in ASU because other wards were full:

Marg Johnson. Broken leg after a nasty fall down the stairs. Husband deceased. No visitors, sadly.

Malcolm Trent. High blood pressure. Severe chest pains.

Fern Barnsley. She was new, I hadn't met her yet. Terrible skin condition, it said. Anyone treating her would require PPE. *Is there even enough available in the cupboard?*

Colin Peters. A chirpy bricklayer, brought in two days prior. Acute bronchitis. Now healing well. Poor thing was placed next to Marg for now. And then . . .

Vivian Butler. Occupation unknown, but a woman well known to the police. A history of taking heroin, but the notes said nothing more.

This was the part of my job I struggled with the most. Medical events and logistics entirely out of my control. Prioritisations of patients no longer made sense: good ones kept waiting too long, bad ones rushed in, undeserving.

A buzzer went off. It came from Colin's bed.

'How are you?' I said, approaching him.

'All the better for seeing you.' He winced, breaking into a fit of coughing. His chest rattled with a deep, dry rhonchi sound. *Look, listen, and feel.* I examined him carefully. His breathing was normal.

I moved to the end of his bed, flicking through his notes: bloods, oxygen respiratory rate and saturation levels, blood pressure. My eyes wearily scanned the squiggly lines and numbers. He'd been given oxygen, antibiotics, steroids and nebulisers. I pulled out a stethoscope and moved closer.

'Lift that a little, would you?'

Colin lifted his T-shirt.

I pressed the chest piece against his skin. 'Sounds like voices echoing in a cave in there.'

His breath quivered. 'Jesus, that's cold.'

'Sorry, I need to check,' I said. 'You've had an X-ray and lung function tests. Everything came back clear. You don't have angina, so that's good. Only bronchitis.'

I stepped back, lowering his T-shirt.

'That's *good*?'

'Bronchitis is treatable. It's not terminal,' I said.

'I suppose there is that.'

A voice interrupted us.

'Yeah, but I wish he'd stop coughing all the time.' Marg lay in the bed opposite. 'Some of us need sleep! It's giving me a bleedin' headache!'

I swung round and walked over to Marg, resisting as much as I could the urge to say what I really felt.

'She's rude, that one,' called Colin. 'Any chance you can move me? She makes me feel worse!'

'No chance,' I said. 'If anything, that bed between you both will be taken. Maybe a new room-mate will help.'

Colin rolled his eyes back.

'Now listen up.' I drew the blue plastic curtains around us and stood over Marg, who was swaddled in a cellular blanket. 'I've heard a few things about you, and I wanted to have a little chat.'

Marg grunted, turning onto her side. Stubbornly, she faced the wall, her back towards me, behaving like a child.

'I've heard you've been saying nasty things to our nurses.'

'Which one?' she muttered. 'They all look the same.'

'Talk like that is offensive, do you understand?'

Marg mumbled expletives under her breath. I moved to the end of her bed to examine her notes. 'This is a verbal warning. Any more of it and we'll have you discharged. It's not something I want to do, but you leave me no choice if you continue.'

She turned, struggling to sit upright. 'I'm in pain, alright?' Marg pulled the sheet off her chest. 'No matter how much I say to that stupid nurse looking after me to go get me more painkillers, she doesn't listen.'

'Maybe she doesn't understand you,' I said.

'Then, for fuck's sake, they should get nurses that speak proper English!'

'You're referring to Anong?' Of course she was. Who else would Marg be talking about? I bit my tongue, trying with all the resolve I had to keep calm.

'I don't know, do I? Don't even know if she's a woman. I'm pretty sure *she's* male. And let me tell you straight: I'm not comfortable being seen by *her* – or *him*. Whatever they call themselves these days.'

I clenched my jaw, my face burning. 'We can't accept discrimination in here. If Anong isn't giving you more medication, it's for a good reason.' I saw in her notes that Marg had already been given a double dose of codeine.

'What discrimination? I'm in need of *treatment*. Paid my taxes and National Insurance my whole life!'

'After a verbal warning comes a written one. If it carries on, we *will* discharge you. Good luck with getting treatment from there onwards.'

Marg dropped her head back onto her pillow. 'Well, just

give me something to die, then, why don't you. Or maybe you don't need to, 'cos at this rate, I will most likely die just lying here . . .'

I emerged from the swish of blue fabric, my heart stuttering and pounding in my chest. I tried to push down my anger to where every negative emotion lived. I reminded myself it wasn't Marg's fault. She was old and frustrated. Pain brought out the worst in people.

I winked at Colin, offering him a consolatory smile. 'If I keep the curtains closed, do you think that will shut her up?'

Colin chuckled, his face round and shining. But then he wheezed, spluttering, grabbing his chest.

'Try not to strain yourself, okay?' I said.

Colin nodded.

I moved to the medical supplies room at the far end of the ward, squeezing the two keys I was authorised to carry as head nurse in my hand. One was to open the main door to the room, the other, the controlled drugs cabinet on the left wall.

Inside, the air was dark and dry. Through a window, a sliver of moonlight emerged from behind a cloud. Around me, dust motes floated, settling onto a small refrigerator on top of the counter. I turned my gaze to the left, to the drugs cabinet, staring at it for a while. I slipped towards the fridge and opened the door. Here, liquid solutions, syrups and elixirs were kept cool. A bottle of antibiotic syrup had leaked, leaving shelves sticky.

I grabbed a packet of antibacterial wipes and began wiping the inside of the fridge. I lifted each bottle, wiping the bottom, neatly replacing it again. When I'd finished, I dried my hands with a cloth, wandering over to the right, glancing up at the hundreds of boxes neatly organised on the shelves. There was the usual selection of painkillers here: aspirin, ibuprofen, co-codamol. But it was morphine, kept in the locked cabinet behind me, that kept calling my name.

My eyes dropped to my feet as temptation rose. I focused on my sensible black shoes, the ladder in my tights snaking around my left ankle. I felt ashamed, terribly ashamed, to give in to weakness like this. Only a few times before had I been tempted to evade detection, helping myself to a handful of tablets, but never once caved in. I'd always managed to rise above it, to think of something else. But today, given the incident with Sandra and now Marg, I was tempted yet again. It was laughable, the cliché of it all. Nurses secretly hooked on morphine, stealing tablets from a locked cabinet in the ward.

I moved to the left wall, turning the key in the lock. Here, I found pregabalin and gabapentin safely tucked at the back. These were used to treat epilepsy, headaches and anxiety. Tramadol, a powerful painkiller related to morphine, would go a long way to melting my aching muscles.

I rummaged around, then pulled out a box, holding it delicately in my hand. I read the label: *100mls of Morphine Oral Solution. 10mg/5ml. Complete with a purple syringe.* I replaced the box and grabbed another. *Morphine Sulphate, Prolonged Release Tablets. 30mg. 10 tablets for oral use.*

In the current climate of overstretch, it would be easy to get away with stealing a strip. I could adjust the ledger, noting down a fake name, date and time, in disguised handwriting. I could scribble a random signature to mirror a day when temp nurses were aplenty. It would work best if I adjusted the notes of a patient about to be discharged, with no follow-up consultation or prescription-check needed afterwards. In this hospital, beds might be in short supply, but drugs were plentiful.

I imagined what it must be like, floating in a blissful haze above the pressure and stress of it all, like drops of oil skittering on the surface of a spring-water lake. But I restrained myself, because no matter how bad things were, I was not like that. I was not like one of those nurses you read about in the papers: struck off for helping themselves to a hospital's medication. I heard a voice inside my head telling me to rise above the temptation, to focus only on compassionate service. Besides, why throw my career away like that after I'd worked so hard to get here?

I bit my lip to stop myself thinking any more about it and locked the cabinet door to continue my shift like a professional.

# 2

I can't tell you how relieved I was to have made it through another night. In this job of relentless service, it's important to acknowledge the little wins as often as you can.

I sent Mercedes a text, reminding her we'd arranged to meet for breakfast. Her shift was about to start, just as mine ended.

We met in the hospital canteen despite the poor quality of food, the toast like cardboard, the tea like dishwater. Mercedes offered to pay – I didn't exactly say no. She had two sources of income. I had just one.

The orange sky of dawn turned into the crisp blue of early morning. Mercedes walked into the hall, bright and breezy, a GUCCI bag slung over her shoulder.

'You look awful,' she said, closely inspecting my face. 'See what happens when you work yourself to death?'

She was full of life, wearing jeans, a sparkly T-shirt. Her curls, tousled springs, bounced over her shoulders. She was more than ready for another round of deliveries in Newgate's maternity unit.

Veering towards the hot-food counter, Mercedes scanned the baked beans, sausages, crispy bacon, then rubbed her hands together enthusiastically. My stomach turned. I couldn't bear the sight of all that grease so soon after my night shift.

'Sorry I haven't been able to call you these past few days. I know we were supposed to meet up,' she said.

'No problem.' I was well used to Mercedes changing plans last minute. 'You going to that community meeting?'

She rolled her eyes. 'Maybe,' she said. 'With all this violence in town, none of us feel safe. Not sure if a community meeting is going to solve it, though.'

'But it's something, at least.'

We selected our food. Mine, a bowl of fruit. For Mercedes, a full English breakfast. 'Yet another reason for me to get out of this shithole,' she said.

We moved to the back of the canteen, balancing our trays and placing them down on a freshly wiped table.

'Here.' Mercedes fumbled around in her handbag, pulling out a pack of cleansing wipes. 'Take this – and oh, here. I got you something . . .' Rummaging further, she pulled it out. 'A blusher. There's a brush inside, see? Saw these on sale and couldn't resist buying them.'

I scanned Mercedes' face, perfectly made up. Like one of those girls you saw in a YouTube make-up tutorial video. I marvelled at how well she seemed to cope with pressure, never appearing to wear the strain of nursing on her face. 'How is it they let you get away with wearing so much make-up?' I said.

'What do you mean, *so much*? Bloody cheek!'

Around me, I scanned the canteen, staff and patients drifting in. 'My shift was pretty full-on,' I said. 'You need to warn the other nurses to be careful.' I grabbed hold of the blusher, prising open the lid.

'What, why?' Mercedes placed her fork down. 'You're scaring me, Nina. What happened?'

I told her about Vivian's attack on Sandra.

'Fucking hell,' she said, sipping her coffee.

'I was more worried about the others, to be honest.' I stared down at the blusher palette, rubbing a finger on the pink blush. 'This is not my colour.'

Mercedes tutted. 'It's neon pink, Nina. *Complementary against dark skin.* It will look great on you. Trust me.' She nudged a packet of cleansing wipes towards me.

I pulled one out, wiping my face down. 'I'm not sure . . .'

'Try it, at least,' Mercedes said. 'So, about Sandra. That is *horrible* – just horrible. She doesn't deserve that. Not when she's just doing her job, checking bloods.'

'Barbara fobbed me off as usual.' I dabbed the brush onto the blush and felt it soft against my cheeks.

Mercedes shook her head, her curls bristling. 'Can't say I'm surprised.' She leaned back into her chair, stretching her arms. 'She's probably right, though. Her hands *are* tied. Not sure how much she can change and influence things.'

*Change and influence.* Such foreign words to me. There wasn't much change and influence you could drive in a system like the one we were in.

Mercedes leaned in closer, whispering. 'What *I'm* hearing is, there's been a mismanagement of funds. That's why the last CEO did a runner – he left a black hole. Richard is doing what he can but it's difficult to fill. So now there's pressure on each department to generate income – to justify themselves. Possibly why Richard insisted on outsourcing bloods to MediCentral, starting with routine and gold standard bloods, but then who knows? Urgent bloods needing a one-hour turnaround next. His bright ideas to save money.'

'Yeah, I heard that as well.'

'The government budget isn't enough. The sooner we get a new PM in office, the better. Maybe then things will be different.'

'But we need more staff now,' I said. I bit into a slice of apple. 'Not sure if that will be Rishi's focus.'

Mercedes cut into a sausage. 'I'm telling you, we're killing ourselves, doing this job. No one is happy about the MediCentral roll-out, what with the ward managers now crawling all over us. I'm counting down the days before I get out.'

I popped a grape into my mouth, chewing slowly because my temples hurt. I placed the blusher palette into my bag. 'Thanks for the make-up. It was sweet of you,' I said.

Mercedes smiled. 'So, speaking of hands tied, Sugar and I went out for dinner.'

I focused on my bowl of fruit. The apples were tired, the grapes, bruised. 'That's nice.'

'Her treat, of course.'

'Of course.'

I wished I had settled for toast.

'We ended up fighting because I told her, I love fancy restaurants, but the portions are a joke!'

'Not enough?'

'Pigeon food, Nina! That's what I call portions like that. I wouldn't mind but they charge an arm and a leg for it. We made up, of course,' said Mercedes quickly, waving a hand in front of her face. 'Our spats are never that deep. You know me, I don't take things too seriously. Not when she's paying.'

I nudged a grape to the side. 'You did once.'

She stopped.

'Remember Jacob? That was serious. You were in love with him.'

She stared at me blankly, blinking twice. 'That was a long time ago,' she said. 'He's gone now. Why d'you bring that up?'

'It's just that . . . things with Sugar. It's all a bit high-maintenance, isn't it? For a longer-term relationship, I mean. She expects you to drop everything without notice. I just worry about you, that's all.'

Mercedes glanced to the side, thinking. 'We have a convenient arrangement, for now. Besides, it's *not* long-term. It pays my bills. I can't live on what they're paying us. I don't know how you do it.'

I glanced down, resolving to grab a plastic box to take my fruit home. 'I budget and keep things simple,' I said.

Mercedes frowned. '*Sensible Nina*.' She took another sip of coffee. 'You off tomorrow?'

'Think so, if the rota doesn't change.'

'Me too. Shall we go and get drunk? I'll do your hair.'

I ran my hand through my hair. 'What's wrong with my hair?'

She smiled. 'Let's forget about Newgate, courtesy of Sugar. She owes me a night out after her fucked-up behaviour. That gives us Friday to recover. Come on. It's not every day we're off together.'

I laughed, because right there was the reason why I'd remained friends with Mercedes for so long. She was like an older sister, living in the moment, always cheering me up.

'Where's good to go on a Thursday night?'

'Electric Blue, Civic Street. We could get there in time for happy hour,' Mercedes said, her eyes glittering. 'If I drink some Red Bull, I could keep going well after my shift.'

I would have had enough sleep, too, I thought. 'Hair and make-up?'

'Sure. I've seen how you put blusher on.' She laughed.

I laughed too. 'But wait. That TikTok video. Aren't you worried?' I said. I stared at her as she searched my face. I'd almost forgotten. 'They threatened something would happen. Not sure we should risk it.' I felt my heart sink a little. There I was, getting all excited, only to realise that going out now was, in fact, dangerous.

'We can't put our lives on hold just because of a gang.' Mercedes shook her head. 'I think we'll be okay.'

That was Mercedes for you. Always willing to take a risk.

We talked, joked and laughed, and as Mercedes stood up to leave, turning to wish me a good night's sleep, I stared out of the window.

A funeral hearse trailed past. A white flower tribute spelled 'MUM', visible through the window.

I grabbed my phone and sent Mercedes a text:

*Thanks for breakfast. See you tonight!*

Mercedes fired a message back:

*Come to mine for 8 p.m. Don't let that stupid video ruin our evening! Xxx*

# 3

The hairstyle Mercedes gave me worked a treat. From the moment I climbed out of the Uber, mid-length hair glamorously puffed and curled, skirt short, heels high, giggling from the several margaritas she'd insisted we down before leaving her flat, all eyes were on me.

I wasn't used to it. Can't say I liked it, even.

But I soon relaxed after several neat vodkas knocked back in the club. Those were swiftly followed by a complimentary tray of tequilas, courtesy of the cool, dreadlocked barman who shuffled and swayed to the music behind the mirrored counter. A crowd of revellers banged their fists as we drank. We made absolute spectacles of ourselves. But by then I didn't care who was watching.

I danced until my feet burned, the chequered floor spinning and whizzing past me in all manner of directions. My throat grew dry from all the cigarettes I'd smoked, which, when plastered with Mercedes, I didn't mind so much.

The next morning, lying in bed with my eyes stuck together, my head throbbing like someone was slamming a sledgehammer against my skull, I discovered there was a man beside me.

I held my breath, gazing at his bare back. Scratches just beneath his shoulder blade made in the dead of night. It was coming back to me, how we'd left the club together.

'Are you awake?' I mumbled, my throat sore.

He stirred and opened his mouth. His tongue clicked as he swallowed. 'What time is it?'

'Two in the afternoon, almost. It's Friday.'

He moved underneath the duvet and sighed.

I stared up at the ceiling, grinning to myself as more recollections of the previous night surfaced like the bubbles in a glass of Prosecco. I saw him leaning against the bar, scanning the dance floor, wearing dark jeans, a black polo shirt. I remembered how I'd sensed the heat fizzing from his body.

By then, Mercedes had left. She'd received an angry text from Sugar to say she had better make herself available once again.

'Do you know what I was thinking when I saw you?' he said as he placed his arm around my waist. Hardly an original line, but I felt myself relax under the blue lights. I let him sway my body to the thrum of the music, and we melted, our bodies melding. 'I was imagining all the things I'd like to do to you.'

An hour later, we stumbled into my flat. He unbuttoned my shirt. His fingers crawled up my back. I hadn't bothered to ask him his name. I suppose I could have asked when I fell back onto the bed, giggling as he unrolled my tights, tugging them at the toes until they slid off my ankles. It just didn't feel like the right moment.

He laughed at the size of my sensible knickers, but stopped when I told him he could fuck off if they weren't the kind of knickers he liked women wearing. He flipped me over; that seemed to mark the end of our talk. He pinned me down, slowly slipping inside but not all the way, at first.

Perhaps anonymity was best.

I glanced at the alarm clock beside my bed. I knew I'd have to make excuses to get him to leave. That TikTok video was still playing on my mind, and there *he* was, in my flat, in my energy field.

'I've got a few things to do,' I said. 'Sorry.'

I glanced around, seeing his clothes scattered across the floor. I'd spent so long tidying up, only for him to be messy.

He rolled over. 'I thought you said you weren't working tonight.'

I saw his face fall. I wasn't sure whether his heart hurt or whether it was his ego.

I heaved myself up onto my elbows. All I kept thinking was, the place needed a jolly good clean. He would have to disappear now, to give me a good few hours to get on with it.

'Nurse, was it?' He tried so hard to remember what we'd said. 'I thought you said you worked nights.'

'I do, but I have some errands. I'm running out of time.'

I climbed out of bed, feeling the comfort of the shaggy pile beneath my feet. I felt him reach out his hand to stroke the curve of my back with his fingertips.

'I was thinking . . .' he said.

The problem with him was that he thought too much.

'I really enjoyed myself and—'

But I hesitated; I hesitated too long.

From the corner of my eye, I watched him stumble out of bed, the smooth of his back, his strong, broad shoulders. He pulled on his polo shirt, then his jeans. His fingers fumbled around the fly for the zip.

The front door closed as the kettle boiled. I was relieved to have gotten rid of him.

I staggered to the sink to brush my teeth. As I prepared breakfast, a part of me felt ashamed. I didn't know why I'd brought a stranger home. To think where he might have been, all those germs and infectious diseases breeding.

Later, there was a knock on the door.

Through the peephole, I saw a man's head, the shiny weave and pleats of his turban. His face was round, jaw neatly bearded. That winning smile was instantly recognisable.

*Balraj.*

He wore a paisley shirt, a waistcoat, a bright-blue scarf. But as I opened the door, I saw his expression downcast. His eyes twitched; his hands fiddled in his pockets.

'Nurse Nina! I am wondering if you are eating something healthy since Diwali is so close.' He held up a clear plastic bag, stuffed with golden samosas.

'It's Diwali on Monday, isn't it? We've still got three days.'

'Yes, yes! You are quite right. But I am never certain of your schedule. I heard you enter last night.' He coughed into his hand, glancing down. He was blushing. 'I did not know you are enjoying nightclubs. I knew you are being at home afterwards . . .'

*This is awkward.*

I opened the door wider to let him in, swallowing down the bile rising. Balraj, my lovable landlord. Though I'd rather not see him right now, how could I refuse him entry? He'd given me a place to live, dead cheap, when I was still a student. Not many would have taken a chance. Next to no money to my name. No references. No guarantee of ever making it through my final nursing exams.

'I will not be long. Just a flying visit to see how you are.'

He entered the flat, glancing over his shoulder like he always did, typical of a landlord about to do a site inspection.

I ran ahead of him, grabbing my knickers off the floor, popping them into the laundry basket.

'You are a very good girl, Nina. Always keeping things clean. I have never seen anyone take so much care of everything.'

I swallowed hard, waiting for his next sentence.

'I could not have a better tenant,' he said.

I moved to the kitchen table, coaxing Balraj to take a seat. I needed to keep a close eye, to understand what he wanted.

'Is that leftovers?' I asked.

'Nothing wasted,' he said cheerfully. 'Balraj is always recycling.'

'Sounds good to me.' Everyone knew the Samosa Hut samosas were famous in Levinstone.

'I am always respecting the traditions of this country. We are closed on Christmas Day, but for Diwali, we are always in service. A good nurse needs much nutrition,' he said, 'and I make my samosas with care and attention.'

He pulled out a chair from under the kitchen table. 'You are coming to the meeting?'

'Wouldn't miss it for the world.'

Balraj glanced down, rubbing his chin. 'Good, good. We must stay positive.' He crossed his legs, and I immediately thought, *here it comes*. His timeless wisdom, a eulogy of some sort.

'When my family came from Jalandhar, Punjab, to try to make a successful business in this country, my father knew –

*absolutely he knew* – it would be very hard work . . .' Balraj circled his finger on the polished tabletop. 'He always said to me "Son, if you work hard, success will come. Good things happen when you invest good energy." And look now! Most likely we will have an Indian prime minister.'

I folded my arms, leaning against the kitchen counter. I suspected I'd be hearing a lot about this, the town so full of South East Asians. Here was a story of immigrant success to believe in, to hold on to even.

'I hope he makes some positive changes, because by God we need it.' I turned, staring down into the sink. My mouth filled with saliva.

'I am always respecting nurses. Do you know, when I had an operation on my back – *terrible pain for five years!* – it is the nurse's face I remember most. Not the doctor.' Balraj winked. 'A pretty girl, just like you. Sheela did not like her.'

I smiled, uncertain how much longer I could keep the bile down. 'I'm sure your lovely wife would be grateful to have you distracted.'

He slapped his thigh and burst out laughing. 'Very naughty girl, you are.' He stopped suddenly and winced. 'Oof!' he said. 'I do not want to remember the pain in my back. *Terrible* it was.'

Balraj uncrossed and crossed his legs, stretching and cracking his fingers.

'The problem is now, young people do not like working hard. Work–life balance, they want. And those youngsters making terrible trouble have no proper ambition. No work ethic.'

I sighed.

'One month in India, then they will learn!'

'Meanwhile, I'm working like a dog,' I said. 'But it's difficult when you don't feel safe or appreciated. People regard us as being nothing more than cleaners. Not that there's anything wrong with being a cleaner.'

'Eh? What are you saying? There is no hospital if there is no nurse. I knew from your eyes when I saw you that day, having nowhere to live, just walking, homeless, near the station. I am thinking, this girl is hungry and lost. I am knowing, *there and then*, you are a good person. God told me to help you. Luckily, I had a flat ready to give you.' He tapped a finger against his temple. 'These days, Balraj is remembering so many things about his life and what he is doing.'

'Well. We need better protection.'

'Say again?'

'Nothing.' I couldn't get into it now. Not so soon after I'd just woken up. But I was thinking of Sandra and the attack. If maybe I was next in line for a punch. 'Would you like some tea, Balraj?' I glanced at the clock. If I made it now and he drank it quickly, he'd be out of here in under twenty minutes. I might still make the meeting.

'You are making?'

I nodded reluctantly, catching sight of the calendar on my cork board where I'd scribbled 'Day off'.

'Then I will not say no.'

He stood up, straightening a pop art print hanging on the wall: Audrey Hepburn surrounded by an explosion of colours. A flat-warming gift from Mercedes who said I should own something modern. All my fluffy cat pictures were making her feel uncomfortable.

Balraj moved to the window, peering onto the pavement below. 'It's getting cold, no?'

'Freezing.'

'And so many terrible robberies and crimes in the area. We are no longer safe, Nina. Not like before. I am feeling uncomfortable. Every night, Sheela is checking the locks on the windows and doors.'

I switched on the gas cooker, heating a pan of water. I knew Balraj wanted Indian tea. Making it was such a palaver.

'Oof! So many pigeons making a mess. Where do they all come from? I wish they would go from here.' Balraj turned. 'Your heating is enough?'

'I try not to use too much.'

'Good, good,' said Balraj. 'Me, also. It is very expensive.'

I approached, handing him a mug of tea. He peered into it, eyes shining, like it was the best thing he'd ever seen.

'Nina . . .'

*Here it comes . . .*

'I must ask you about the rent,' he said. 'I know you are working very hard. But rent must be paid on time.'

I felt my stomach twinge, my cheeks flush. 'I'm sorry. I forgot. It must have slipped my mind with everything going on.' I felt so stupid and yet I knew I'd deliberately held it back. When there's so little money to play with, it's only natural to want to hold on to it for as long as you can. But I regretted it now. The last thing I wanted was to let Balraj down. 'I'll do a transfer now, in front of you, so you know it's done.'

I placed my mug down, a splash of tea spilling onto the counter. I grabbed my laptop, sliding it out of its felt cover.

I logged into my account as quickly as my fingers could key in the digits.

'Take your time, take your time,' he said. 'I am feeling embarrassed asking you, but you understand, yes? If people are helping you with good discount, rent must still be paid on time.'

'Of course. Don't apologise. It's my fault.'

'It's very important.'

'Yes, Balraj.'

'Actually, when they are helping you, it is *more* important not being late.'

'So sorry, once again.'

I felt my stomach clench more tightly. I was stupid, fucking stupid, to ever treat a man who had been generous to me like this.

My account popped up on screen and I viewed my balance. I furiously scanned the numbers crawling around like insects. A long chain of debits, one measly credit. I had enough to pay the rent, eight hundred pounds, but there was not much left over to see me through the rest of the month.

'I'm doing you a transfer now,' I said.

*Balance: fifty pounds.*

I bit the inside of my cheek and slammed my laptop closed. 'And your lovely wife? How is her health?'

'Sheela is okay. Just a little sad. But still, she is giving me a big headache. Always changing furnishings. It is unnecessary, I say. Please, stop wasting money! No need for different bedclothes every month. We are in a cost-of-living crisis. Too many nice things will mean people will rob us!'

But by now, I struggled to listen. My mind was ticking, performing mental calculations. I scrambled to figure out how I would cover my expenses. There was travel and food. Bus tickets were cheaper than petrol. I'd have to reduce my use of the car. That was okay because my car was, at best, unreliable – the suspension, about to pack in. I didn't have enough money to take it to the garage. Plus, parking was so expensive after the hospital management got rid of the subsidy for staff.

'Well, I must go now.' Balraj stood up, placing his empty mug down. 'Happy Diwali to you. I hope you stay healthy. This new year is very special to us Asians.'

'It is?' I mumbled. 'You know I'm half, so I'm not too bothered.'

'Of course! But half is still half. I can see on which side you are.' He came closer, patting me on the back. 'You are more Indian, yes? I see it in your face and in your behaviour.'

It took me back a little to hear him say that, but I supposed it was true. That part of myself was something I could, at least, hold on to. I might not have felt like one of them, but the story of Asian success, of good immigration, was positive, at least. What did the other side bring? Unconscious bias, negative stereotypes: gangs, drugs, the constant threat of violence. Not knowing who I was, I had to choose. Of course, I would be lying if I didn't admit that later, I would live to regret my ignorance.

At the front door, I waved Balraj off. But as he climbed down the stairs, he stopped and turned.

'I want you to be happy, Nina. Any problem, you come

and see me. Balraj is here for you. One day you will make a man very happy. I am certain of it.'

I scoffed. 'What makes you think I want to get married?' I preferred my own company, couldn't he tell? Some of us were lone wolves. Born in the wild, always scavenging for food.

Balraj shook his head. 'Oof!' he said. 'You must not say such things. You are enjoying your life; I will not judge it. But one day you will want a good husband.'

I closed the door, listened to it clunk. Then ran to the kitchen sink to violently throw up.

# 4

In Christ Our Redeemer Community Church, red velvet chairs were arranged theatre-style. I entered, straightening my skirt, painfully aware of just how late I was. Eyes followed me as I scrambled for a space somewhere in the middle, on the aisle.

'Despite threats of criminal intent on social media, there's no fixed date mentioned. This might all be a sick joke, intended to attract attention.'

DC Barry Coombs stood at the front on a makeshift stage. Microphone in hand, he looked like a DJ in a kid's primary-school disco. 'Of course, we're doing what we can to prepare. It's all we can do right now.'

Pastor Oswald Otis was at the front. I wondered if this was his way to 'outreach', to prove to secular folk that God still existed.

I scanned the audience, warmed by the cultural mix in the crowd. Another reminder of why I loved Levinstone. There were whites, a few East Asians, the majority West African and Caribbean. Next, South Asians. I noticed a handful of Eastern Europeans too, but mainly they kept to themselves.

Pastor Otis stared thoughtfully into space, hands clasped, moving lips as if whispering the Lord's Prayer.

An elegant arm shot up from somewhere in the middle.

'So, what exactly *are* the police doing to prepare, because lack of assurance from *you* is what's provoked the convening of this meeting in the first place.' That was Farah Khan, a local reporter. Worked for the *Levinstone Gazette.* I'd heard she was pushy, sensationalising local news to click-bait national attention.

'Well . . .' Barry shifted his weight. 'The police are looking into known agitators, aggressors – anyone we think might be potential suspects. Rest assured, we've a plan to mobilise forces quickly in the event of an incident. But right now, no crime has been committed.'

There were groans in the hall. The crowd grew unsettled. Some tutted, kissing their teeth. Others waved their hands with agitation.

Barry formed part of a five-strong panel of local representatives from each service area: education, social services, the local health service, and the police. Neighbourhood Watch were there, too; they'd organised the meeting.

'Why can't you just arrest them based on their threats – looking at their social media profiles?' That was Derek; his question was fair. He ran a local newsagent but carried himself like a cartoon detective. 'Surely, you've got teams in place to deal with that sort of thing. You can contact the online platforms themselves – TikTok, Facebook – to trace account holders.'

Barry's face flushed, affronted by the insinuation that he didn't know how to do his job. 'Online threats are still real and constitute a criminal offence. Those posts come from one account, and we *will* arrest on the back of it. If we manage to track down the account holder, that is.'

Voices murmured; the air grew thick with questions.

I scanned the crowds and was surprised to spot Richard

Lonsdale, Newgate Hospital's CEO, sitting in the corner. Presumably he was here to make a point of showing support. He was tall and thin with protruding cheekbones. His face strained as he listened.

None of what I was hearing sat particularly well with me. I rather liked living in Levinstone and didn't want to feel unsafe here. *As long as those threats don't turn real,* was all I kept thinking. I didn't want those thugs finding their way into Newgate, either.

I scanned the hall and wondered if out there, somewhere in the crowd, were their parents.

'We're dealing with sophisticated individuals, part of a gang, or several gangs teaming up,' Barry said. 'They've gone to great lengths to conceal their identity. We've no affirmative details of their plans. We're exploring all methods of intelligence available to us.'

I glanced at a trestle table pushed against the wall. Biscuits, teas, plantain and cassava chips were laid out. There was an oil-smudged box labelled 'Vegetable Samosas'. Next to it, someone had baked fresh banana bread. My stomach rumbled. I grabbed a serviette and a samosa, piling on cassava chips.

'Regardless, you have our assurance,' said Barry, 'that we're doing everything we can to keep things safe. Anyone caught breaking the law *will* be arrested.'

I sat back down, munching as I listened. For weeks now, I'd heard the same thing. Those in authority, positions of power, extending their sorry excuses for things going downhill. This was my home. Only those who have grown up without one will know how much that means to a person.

I didn't want people sitting back, twiddling their thumbs. I wanted them to get up and to *do* something.

My arm shot up, I cleared my throat.

'I'm Nina, a nurse at Newgate Hospital.' Heads turned in my direction. With everything going on, I wanted to say my bit. But somehow, with all eyes on me, I felt intimidated. I scrunched the serviette and balled my fist. 'Some of us work nights because, well . . . we have no choice and need the money.'

People nodded, offering compassionate understanding. With their support, it didn't matter to me that Richard was watching.

'The way things are going, we don't feel safe travelling to work. Also . . .' I looked around me. 'All this *crime* on our streets is tragic. This is our home. We must protect it. I don't feel like we're doing enough. I hate to say it . . . but there are some in this community that don't deserve to be here.'

Barry stared at me, perplexed, an expression hard to read. I wasn't having a go at the police, but I didn't mind him taking it personally.

'We need to find a way to bring back what was once great about this place,' I said, 'to keep ourselves safe. This town was alive once, before the pandemic ruined things. The history of the area, if people can be bothered to look it up, is of civil action. Youth-led movements in the sixties and seventies. National campaigns against racism, safer buildings. There were factory lines. Textile wholesalers . . . We should be rebuilding this community, together.'

The crowd nodded.

'I know we're meeting about a specific online video threat, but we all know we're experiencing increased crime rates. We shouldn't have to change our lives. It's the bad people that do bad things that need to get the hell out of here.'

People clapped. I realised how good that felt.

I sat down, breathing heavily, my knees weak. I was proud of myself for speaking out.

Next to me, a woman in a pink tracksuit raised her hand.

'We need answers about what to do. If nurses are scared, talking about punishment, you know it's serious.'

'It's out of control,' a woman called from the back. Her voice slashed the air like a knife. Smartly dressed, she looked like she worked in a branch of Lloyds Bank on the high street. She stood up, straightening herself. 'My name is Manisha, and what *I* think is that there's no excuse for this antisocial behaviour. In the land of free education there is plenty of opportunity and access. I have a son and, believe me, I am strict with him. Parents should instil the right values in their children.'

Balraj was sitting to my left, two rows in front. He nodded in emphatic agreement, whispering to a woman wrapped in a red scarf pinned with a lizard brooch.

A man with a ginger beard stood up. 'She's right. I run the off-licence on Civic Street and what *I* think is that we're living in the land of the lawless. Burglaries, stabbings, shootings. Threats of looting and more violence. We've seen the same happening in America, and now it's happening over here, and we don't want it!'

'Hear, hear!' I shouted.

Neighbourhood Watch wittered on about the need for a

more harmonious community, then a rep from education talked about longer-term strategic interventions. What none of them were saying was that most of those criminals were assumed to be black or brown. I knew what some folks were thinking. Why they'd ever let control slip in this town. But I had mixed emotions, too. These youths were feeding that prejudice. And there I was, slap bang in the centre of those two sides, listening to excuses for how some kids downward spiral, lacking this or that.

As far as I was concerned, I *also* had a hard life, a terrible upbringing which I dared not talk about. But I turned out just fine. Someone ought to tell them: crime was a choice, not a medical condition.

'You need to remember, essential investment has been cut, libraries, parks, youth centres . . . Where do these kids go when a system has failed them?'

Thoughts of the previous night hit me. I swallowed hard.

A man from the back shouted in a gruff voice. 'But we have shit happening all over town so we need to focus on what you're gonna do about it, *now*!' A cluster of heads turned. 'They ride BMXs for Christ's sake! They're not that hard up!'

Another woman stood up. 'Nina the nurse is right . . .'

My ears pricked.

'We don't feel safe leaving our homes. And they're getting younger, that's true. But you all need to understand that this issue is complex.'

I could see her supporters nodding.

'My name is Grace . . .' Her face was wide like a broadsheet, her expression a tragic headline. 'I'm a local primary schoolteacher.'

For some, recognition descended.

'From talking to my son, familiar with such groups, I understand these youngsters are frightened themselves. That's why they carry knives and lash out. What they're doing is protecting themselves.'

Barry grabbed hold of the microphone. 'Grace is right . . . many of these youths are simply children themselves. They are more likely to be stabbed by their own knife than anyone else's. We need to understand, they are afraid and vulnerable.'

I wasn't sure whether the two of them knew each other, or whether their tag-team approach was merely a coincidence.

Grace nodded, appreciative of the support.

Barry switched off the microphone, placing it on the table.

Pastor Oswald Otis shook his foot nervously, then stood up and shouted, 'Praise the Lord!' Around him, some of his supporters raised their hands and joined in the chant.

It was complex, all this. I wondered whether, thinking only of myself, I had been selfish. I'd attended this meeting because of concerns for my own safety. It didn't occur to me that perpetrators of the problem might need support as well.

Around us, people weren't sure what to do with themselves. The meeting had ended suddenly without a clear outcome. I remained in my seat as people stood, chattering, chairs scraping. They began dispersing, ushered by Pastor Oswald Otis to try some of the international feasts on offer. Leaflets were handed out, encouraging everyone to post their views in an online community forum: www.levinstonematters.com.

Farah remained, scribbling on her notepad. Later, I would recall that scene of her often. How we'd first met. How I should have known her real intention then. But in that moment, I simply wondered how she'd made reporting news her living. Whether a woman like Farah had answers to our problems.

I watched as she slipped her notebook and pen into her back pocket. She stood up and sauntered to the table. Cool, centred, she eyed up the Nongshim Shin cup noodles.

I followed behind, trying to be discreet.

Balraj waved, and I waved back. Farah turned, sizing me up and down. She moved closer. 'Why do I feel like I've seen you before?' she said, peering at me.

*I need coffee and I need it now.*

'I'm Nina, a nurse at Newgate. You might have seen me there,' I said.

She nodded. 'I'm Farah, reporter for the *Levinstone Gazette*. Cover mostly crime.' She offered her hand.

'I know.' Her hand felt fleshy and cold as I shook it. 'We've all read your articles.'

She tore the foil lid off the cup noodles and smiled. 'Well, that's good to hear. Nice to know I'm writing something relevant. My editor does like to carefully curate.' She glanced around her and sighed. 'Doesn't seem to understand that local stories are fine, but it's national attention that's needed to drive systemic change.'

She poured hot water on her noodles, jabbing her fork in the mound.

'What stories are you covering now?' I asked, genuinely interested.

'Stabbings, shootings, robberies – that sort of thing.' She glanced up at the stained-glass window. 'A few cases of fraud and scamming; that seems to be growing.'

I thought what a joy Farah's job must be, to write about stories from a distance without ever having to live through them.

'I'm looking for something big, though.' Her face turned, eyes narrowing. 'You work at Newgate, did you say?' She blew over her fork, shoving crispy noodles into her mouth.

'Been there five years,' I said.

'Interesting.' She placed a hand over her lips. 'I'd love to talk to you about what's going on there,' she said, chewing. Her eyes had lit up.

'About what, exactly?'

'Hospitals are pressure cookers, aren't they? We all know there's stuff going on inside.' She glanced around her, catching sight of Richard pouring coffee. 'New CEO. Lots of changes.'

'I don't know what you're talking about,' I said, because really, I didn't. Not then, at least.

'There's probably a lot that doesn't get talked about. Good to get a bit of inside information.'

She was persistent, I had to give her that.

I was half tempted to indulge her, but I sensed Richard watching me from the corner. He stood next to Barry, and they struck up a conversation. 'We're not allowed to talk to the press. It's in our contracts,' I said.

Farah nodded, shoving more noodles into her mouth. Watching her eat made me salivate. I glanced at the table longingly, at the cassava chips, and grabbed a few more.

'Well, you know where I am if you want to talk.' Farah

dabbed her mouth on the sleeve of her jumper. Barry stood in the corner on his phone. 'I don't think they'll continue the panel discussion. It just winds people up.'

'I'd better go,' I said. 'Maybe next time.' Her work was worthwhile, but I didn't want to get involved in it.

'Wait! I've got a card. Let me go grab it—' Farah placed her noodles down on the counter.

But I was gone.

Outside it rained. I pulled my coat tightly around me, covering my neck. Just as I was about to leave the courtyard, I heard someone calling after me.

I turned and saw it was Richard, waving from the entrance.

'Was hoping to catch you,' he said, walking towards me. I wasn't sure what to do or say. We'd never spoken. 'Just wanted to say hello. I think I've seen you in the hospital.'

I smiled awkwardly, an attempt to be polite. I couldn't take my eyes off Richard's leather-like face. 'I'm nurse in charge in Florence Nightingale.'

'Ah! That must be it,' he said, nodding. 'I thought you looked familiar. Terrible situation, all this. I'm glad I attended to fully understand it.' He peered at me. 'Things are well with you? You're enjoying your job?'

'Sure, I love working at Newgate,' I said coyly.

'Great to hear.' He pressed the handle of his umbrella, holding it over me like the proper gentleman he appeared to be. Well mannered. Educated. 'Many exciting times ahead.'

For a second, I stood awkwardly, wanting to keep our conversation short. He was the hospital CEO, driving through change. I felt small in his presence.

'Would you like a lift home? This rain is rather inconvenient.' Richard closed his umbrella. 'My car's just over there.'

A black Jaguar was parked on the kerb.

'I'm alright. I'll take the bus – it's quicker.'

'Very well. Hope to see you at Newgate!' He waved as he trotted off.

I watched him climb into his car, listening to the sound of his engine purr like a well-fed cat. He turned the wheel to pull out. A flock of pigeons cooed and flew ahead of us. As the last pigeon rose, a waft of powdery grey, something on the lonely street lay empty and unsaid. *When those who are meant to care for you discard you like a dirty rag, this town, your only home, is all that's left to love.*

I knew I had to play my part in trying to protect this town. A home is where it begins, a home is where it all ends. I would surely kill to keep it safe.

# 5

I stared into my near-empty fridge. Leaning an arm on the open door, I pulled out whatever there was – two carrots, a wilting half cabbage – and placed them on the counter. My phone vibrated in the back pocket of my jeans. I stared at the number flashing and swiped to answer it.

'Nina, it's Barbara . . .'

Hearing her voice, strained and panting, took me back.

'I feel terrible calling you on your day off.'

'I've just got back from the community meeting,' I said. 'How can I help?'

'We've got a few illnesses . . . There appears to be a bug going around . . .'

My heart sank.

'I wondered if you wouldn't mind coming in to do a shift. I'm sorry to have to ask you. Platinum Care are struggling to send someone.'

I thought of Balraj, of having just paid the rent. With the extra shift came a little more money to cover the essentials. I didn't think twice, though I desperately wanted the time off.

'I can be there at eight as usual,' I said. I checked my watch. By now it was almost six o'clock.

'You could? Oh, Nina. I'm ever so grateful. The usual start is fine.'

I placed my phone on the counter; the loud hum from the open fridge pierced through me like a sinister laugh. It ridiculed my utter stupidity for thinking I could enjoy an evening off.

On the bus, I tapped my Oyster onto the pay disc and staggered up the narrow stairwell to the upper deck. I clutched on to the handrails for dear life as the bus took off. Collapsing into my seat, I sent Mercedes a text:

*Last night was fun! We need more nights like that. They called me in – can you believe it? On my way now. Bus is carnage! xx*

Mercedes sent a text back:

*Oh that is rubbish!! I'll catch you in Newgate tomorrow! So sorry you have to work* :( *Xxx*

I must have grown distracted, staring at a couple talking to one another in front, their exchanges growing heated when they began discussing Christmas plans. I barely noticed the bus halting, just past the town hall, where the council's main office was. The driver announced he wouldn't take a risk and drive us any further.

I looked out of the window, wondering what the hell was going on.

Outside, crowds gathered. They were shouting, screaming. A short, sharp hiss and the bus lowered. The engine switched off.

The driver yelled, 'Everyone stay in your seats! I'm keeping the doors closed for your safety!'

My heart began thumping hard.

Set back from the main road, on a corner outside Screaming Motors – an auto-repair garage that had fleeced me on at least two separate occasions – young men on BMXs in black puffers coalesced. There must have been at least thirty of them of different races – black, white, Asian, mixed. Hoods pulled up, so you couldn't see their faces.

I remembered the threats from the TikTok video and switched my phone to camera mode.

The wheels screeched as they braked. The men slung their bikes onto the pavement. They climbed off, forming a large group, nodding, sharing secret signals. I'd seen so many of them in town, most of them loud, smoking joints on street corners, playing music, sweary and offensive. Most likely murderous too. We'd seen the effects of their muggings, stabbings, lootings, heard all about it in the community meeting.

They ambled as if waiting.

Though not all of them were black, sure as hell, it would be black men shouldering the blame. It was precisely why I leaned towards the more Asian side of me. Less likely to stir and rile. Less likely to get into trouble.

This was it. This must be the raid.

They shouted and nudged one another to go on and enter the garage.

I pictured the poor mechanics inside, cowering in fear, too scared to emerge from under their bonnets. Some of the young men carried weapons: batons, knives, that sort of thing. I didn't see any guns, however.

More men appeared – ones wearing red puffers. Presumably

from Lyndon Hill, the neighbouring town. An argument developed, each gang staring the other out. They hissed and spat, ready to pounce. Some of them rushed into Screaming Motors. In the scuffle, a few men collided at the entrance. I wasn't sure who, which side, but I thought I heard a yell. A man shouted for them to get the hell out of the way, to go and get proper jobs.

I pressed REC as arms went up, as a rain of red fists came pelting down. I could tell from the screams of passers-by, watching in horror and disbelief, scrambling to stand at a safe distance, that this was an assault on an innocent civilian. Someone had collapsed on the floor. That poor *someone*, the object of this gang's aggression, paying the price for simply daring to confront them.

I stood up unsteadily, my phone in one hand, my bag in the other. I saw only the victim's shoes: faded brown leather loafers, soles scuffed, the tips coming apart at the toes.

A woman on the bus screamed.

Downstairs, the driver scrambled out of his seat. Fists were thumping on the door.

My hand shook. I zoomed in on a bright-blue scarf strewn on the pavement. It was just about visible through a triangle-shaped gap between a man's thick legs sporting white joggers. Impossible to make out the victim's face. The camera lens focused and refocused because I was so unsteady.

Swarming like flies around the body were the boys, red and black hoods now mixed up and slipping to their necks. Balaclavas, bandanas, crowned with the initials SK and LH. The letters of the two rival gangs we all recognised.

That man in white joggers, whom I saw was black, now straightened up. From the way he moved, he appeared jittery and nervous. He looked young, no older than twenty, wearing a chunky gold bracelet hanging over what looked like a barbed-wire tattoo needled around his wrist.

He kept himself at a distance from the others, twitching about the victim, glancing left, right, and then behind him. He wore designer trainers, the holograms on the sides glistening.

As realisation dawned that everyone was filming on their phones, he made a point of covering his face, shouting to the other boys in black hoodies to do the same. They shot up, as if standing to his command. 'I said it's done, yeah? Let's get the fuck out!'

A herd of police officers came running down the street carrying spray gas, batons, plastic shields. On the bus, people clambered to get a better view. They held their phones higher, screens pressed flat against the glass. A man next to me slid open the upper pane of the window to capture better sound.

People chanted 'Is he dead, is he dead?' But all I kept thinking was, if he's dead, that would mean murder. Next must follow a big police investigation.

I stopped filming and replaced my phone in my bag. My head rushed at the thought that I might have captured vital evidence about the criminals destroying this town.

There was a crashing noise, like a metal bin falling over. I looked up. The man in the white joggers was screaming into his phone. For a second, he stopped; his face shot up, eyes menacing, as if something dark had glazed over them. They pierced into me with an incredible power and focus.

I watched him climb onto his bike, pedalling fast to escape the scene. His silhouette minimised on the horizon as more police in vans appeared.

The roar of the engines and sirens was deafening.

I let out a long breath, my limbs rubbery and numb, and collapsed into my seat. My chest heaved, heart beating so hard, I thought I might be sick. To my left, through the window, I saw the few remaining men straggling, unsure what to do with themselves. They were without bikes, now walking fast, trying to act normal. They ran when the police chased after them. Thrown to the ground, their arms stretched, hands cuffed firmly behind their backs, some were arrested and thrown into vans.

The bus fired up its engine. As the commotion settled down, everyone returned to their seats, staring at the pavement below. I struggled to process what I'd witnessed. That poor man was still there, his body crumpled, a pool of blood trickling onto the kerb. Six paramedics were there too, one kneeling beside him, frantically pumping his chest, others helping to lay out a stretcher for the ambulance.

I was numb by the time I got into work. I turned over what happened in my mind, the gaze of those eyes still boring into me. I didn't want to talk, only to carry out whatever tasks were mandatory. But it was not easy to forget the sight of that poor man left dying on the pavement.

# 6

At the nurse's station in Florence Nightingale ward, I snatched a cup from the water cooler. The cold shocked my teeth as I gulped. My throat constricted as I swallowed.

I felt a tap on the shoulder and swung round.

It was Maria. 'Everything okay? Just checking in.'

I nodded. 'I'm fine. Why would you ask?' I wondered whether my behaviour had revealed too much.

'Just wanted to make sure, what with the new Medi-Central roll-out for bloods. There's a lot going on. All of it urgent, it seems.' She sighed.

'I'm aware,' I said, curter than I'd intended.

'And you're absolutely clear on new procedures? Though Richard's insisted we implement in earnest, we still can't have any errors. It's important this goes well.'

'Of course.' Always the professional. 'Down separate chutes, urgent versus routine. Gold standard tests clearly labelled and prioritised,' I said.

Maria smiled. 'Thanks, Nina. You're always so reliable.'

I nodded, clenching my jaw as Maria turned on her heels and walked off. I didn't have too much time to think because the phone rang. Seeing that red light flicker on the phone base made my breath catch. I remembered the flash of the police sirens, the ambulance.

I picked up the handset, pressing it close to my ear. 'Nurse Nina,' I breathed.

I could still see, when I closed my eyes, that sight – that scramble, from the bus.

'Hello, goddess.'

'Jimmi . . .' My stomach twinged.

'Don't say my name like that.'

'Like what?

'Like you're describing the symptoms of gonorrhoea.'

Jimmi Rangoon was a bed and site manager, overseeing hospital logistics. By his own admission, that made him powerful. One night, after a few glasses of cheap wine, he'd shown he had a certain appeal. Though he was a little shabby, in need of a good haircut, chest puffed out like a baked potato with too much of his own crude talk and self-importance, I admit, I had been lonely.

I glanced up at the clock on the wall surrounded by Post-its and thank-you cards. 'Make it quick,' I said. 'I'm busy. Had a terrible start to the evening. I'm not even supposed to be here.'

He paused. 'That's not very nice, Nina.'

'Just saying.'

He cleared his throat. 'I've got a couple in A&E.' His voice was harder, more professional. 'One with terrible stomach pains. Another with stab wounds. Both have been triaged but need further treatment. All yours if you're interested.'

I scrolled through patient files on my PC, clicking my mouse deliberately loudly so that Jimmi could hear the efforts I was making. 'No room here, I'm afraid.' I just couldn't face dealing with them.

He paused. 'What? Impossible. You should have two beds, that is unless that bloody idiot Sunil from IT has not been keeping our systems updated. Honestly, despite my complaints, everything is so clunky. Like my job isn't hard enough.'

'I can't help you,' I said, biting my lip as my mouth filled with saliva. 'We don't have enough beds or nurses. At least not in *this* ward.'

Jimmi said he needed to think. That he hadn't expected me to say that, and it had thrown him. I imagined him scrolling through admissions, trying to see how he'd made a mistake.

'If you're sure . . .'

'I'm sure,' I said.

It was wrong of me to lie. Of course, looking back now, I *know* that. But at the time, I thought, *This is Jimmi.* He knew as well as I did; we simply couldn't cope. I needed to create space so that we nurses could do our jobs better.

I left it like that, hanging up. Hoping I wouldn't be found out. But just as I was about to turn my back, the phone rang once more.

'Numbers don't add up, Nina.'

*Jimmi.*

'I hope you're not messing about. That would be unethical.'

'What will you do, arrest me?' I laughed. I placed the handset down, my hand trembling.

I stayed at the front desk for another ten minutes, but through the glass doors I saw Jimmi approaching. My stomach clenched tight like a fist. I kept my head bowed, scribbling random words onto a piece of paper to make it look like I was busy.

I shouldn't care, not after Vivian's attack on Sandra, the blood I'd seen trickling down the pavement. But Jimmi stepped forward, leaning his weight over the ledge.

'See this here?' he said, holding up a printout. 'What I don't understand is that *this* states, clearly, "Two beds available, Florence Nightingale".' He turned, scanning the ward. 'You'd better make arrangements for them to be transferred, pronto.'

I looked down. 'The notes are a mess. It was an honest mistake. No need to get your knickers in a twist over it.'

Jimmi narrowed his eyes, then laughed out loud. 'It's bad karma to be horrible during Diwali, so I'll let you off. Better not let it happen again, though. If it wasn't *me* in charge, serious questions would be asked.'

I began to grow weary of the time, impatience thinning my blood like warfarin. 'Who have we got?' I said. 'Let's get it over and done with.'

'First up, Dev Shah. Aged twenty. Bad stomach pains. Needs a quiet corner.'

Barbara rushed past, a folder wedged under her arm. Maria followed closely behind her.

'Second, Leroy Sanchez. A bit more complex.'

I searched for a pen, my physical movements one step behind the ticking going off inside my brain. It was my night out with Mercedes catching up with me. I was overcome by a sudden feeling of exhaustion.

'Can you slow down a bit? Dev Shah. How bad is it?' I allocated Dev to Florence Nightingale, despite everything.

'Bad, I think. He's got loose bowels, but probably not as bad as the diarrhoea I had after my holiday in Thailand.'

Jimmi chuckled. 'Did I tell you about that?' For some unknown reason, he felt it was appropriate to mention it.

I prepared Dev's notes, saw he'd already had standard blood tests – an FBC, full blood count. He'd been tested for a list of other things too: U&Es, urea and electrolytes, plus LFTs – liver function tests – a clotting screen and CRP – reactive protein check. He'd even had an amylase to exclude pancreatitis. But his pain persisted – no one could figure it out. Central then right on his lower abdomen. Tenderness combined with a fever. They'd said, owing to slightly high CRP and WBC counts, an appendicectomy would be worth doing. But his notes didn't say he had appendicitis, only that it was suspected.

'Give me twenty to sort him out,' I said.

'Great.'

'And Leroy, did you say?'

'Leroy Sanchez. Part of a gang of four. Suffering a stab wound.'

My chest tightened.

'*Four?*'

'We're taking them all in for twenty-four hours. Strict orders. They've been separated. You're taking Leroy after he's been stitched up in theatre. The other three, I need to sort, still.'

I scanned down the ward's admissions and flinched.

'Do they have anything to do with the raid? I feel very uncomfortable about treating them. I was there, on the bus. I saw the whole thing . . .'

'Part of the Stone Killaz,' said Jimmi, grinning. He moved his fingers, signing the letters, SK.

'That's not funny,' I said.

'Chill, Nina! He'll be escorted and supervised by the police.'

'Hardly reassuring. Can't he go elsewhere?'

'We've got to take them all in,' said Jimmi, 'we're the NHS, remember. Criminals, mass murderers, paedophiles. Free democratic healthcare for all.'

'I'm not happy about this,' I said, as I prepared Leroy's notes. The knife had not hit a vital organ so his time in theatre would be short.

'I won't lie,' said Jimmi, relishing the fear in my face. 'They've been known to use extreme violence – acid sprays, imitation arms, setting dangerous dogs onto victims. Just the usual stuff that goes on around here. Plus, the expected stabbings. These days it's not safe for a woman to be out on her own, know what I mean? Good to have a man around.'

I was perspiring, my scrubs sticking to my back.

'You have my personal number . . .' Jimmi glanced up at the clock. 'If you have time, that is.' He smiled. 'Happy Diwali, Nina. I've got a feeling this new year is going to be a good one.'

Jimmi walked to the door and I traipsed behind him, even pressing the exit button to help shuffle him out of the ward. When I returned to the nurse's station, my head hung heavy in thought.

The buzzer went off again, and as I looked up, I saw a man's face through the glass.

It was a porter I hadn't seen before, which was strange because I knew all of them. He must be new. I could just about make out his face, his square jaw, sculpted cheekbones. A Teutonic profile topped with messy brown hair. But there was something about the way he moved – gliding almost, etheric, other-worldly – that suspended my intense interest.

I pressed the buzzer to let him in. He wheeled in a patient I assumed must be Dev. So much for giving me twenty minutes.

A woman shuffled behind him.

'Are you Mum?' I asked. I walked towards her, realising I'd seen her at the community meeting. Her face was sunken and lost, her eyes puffy and dark-circled. Her hair was messily scraped back, twisted into a bun with loose tendrils tumbling at the sides to hide her stick-out ears.

She lifted her glasses, dabbing her eyes with a tissue. 'My name is Manisha.'

I glanced down at Dev, wondering what it must be like to have been brought up on his mother's *good values*.

'It's you,' she said. She appeared to recognise me, too.

'Don't worry. We'll take care of him as best as we can.'

I glanced at the porter and smiled, noticing a flash of something in his eyes, warm and green. An invitation, it seemed.

'I haven't seen you before,' I said, admiring his face. His skin was pale, translucent. Not necessarily attractive in the conventional sense. But there I was, staring at him all the same.

'I'm Nikolaus,' he said, smiling.

Dev lay under a white sheet, a blue cellular blanket thrown over him.

I placed my hand on his arm, glancing at his knees tucked to his stomach. 'My name is Nina Dabral. I'm a nurse here.

I'll be taking care of you while the doctor arrives to further examine you.' He swallowed and nodded. I glanced up at Nikolaus and caught him staring at me. My body flushed as he quickly looked away.

'My mum . . . she's worried,' Dev said. 'But I'm alright, aren't I? Tell her I'll be fine. Just need . . . the operation.'

'You'll be on your feet in no time,' I said, taking in his face: neat and round with boyish features.

I squeezed Manisha's shoulder. 'He'll be fine, don't worry. We'll get to the bottom of whatever it is that's causing him trouble.' I flicked through his notes. 'The appendectomy will help. Time to be confirmed, still.'

She nodded.

The wheels of the trolley rattled as Nikolaus and I steered Dev. Colin and Marg were asleep. Gently, we grabbed the end of the bed and manoeuvred him into the small space between them.

Dev leaned to one side, a hand covering his damp face. I pulled the plastic curtains closed; they billowed in the breeze of our movements. I wanted to urgently carry out the necessary obs, blood pressure, pulse, oxygen saturations, respiratory rate. The usual temperature checks.

I kicked the trolley's brake, noticing Nikolaus's strong arms, the tattoos of snakes and skulls. Something about them, in this heated moment, this pressured environment, felt strangely sexual.

I rearranged my hair. 'Hopefully, you'll feel a bit more relaxed here,' I said to Dev, watching Nikolaus from the corner of my eye, the way he ran a hand along his thigh. 'You've got a comfortable spot at least.'

'That's something,' said Manisha. She took a seat on the visitor's chair. 'It's the first time I'm resting my feet. We waited *ages* in A&E – they've no sense of urgency. Just getting test results took hours.'

I took Dev's temperature, placing the probe under his tongue, making a note of it. 'You're thirty-eight degrees, which is very high. Have you drunk any water?'

Dev shook his head.

I checked his blood pressure, wrapping a cuff around his arm, then his heart and respiratory rates. All three, a little high.

'I'll grab a cold towel to cool you down,' I said. 'I'll try and get a doctor to see you as soon as I can.'

Manisha covered her face with her hands, and I went to fetch a flannel. I was thinking of Nikolaus, how that sight of him had lifted me a little. But when I checked on waiting times, I saw it was longer than usual.

I returned after a minute, the flannel soaking wet in my hands. 'Current waiting time is five hours,' I said. 'I'm terribly sorry. It's very busy tonight.'

I noticed Nikolaus was gone.

'Five hours?' gasped Manisha.

This was the part I struggled with the most, allocation and waiting times, entirely out of my control.

'We're flat-out,' I said, pressing the flannel onto Dev's forehead. 'But it's still nil by mouth and no fluids for two hours. You could be called any minute. Says in the notes we need to run more blood tests too – gold standard. I'll ask for a rush service of one hour so you don't have to wait too long for results. Or at least, that's the hope. I'll also administer

IV fluids and antibiotics in the meantime, and keep chasing for the doctor.'

'Another blood test?' I felt Manisha's exasperation like a stab in the neck. 'We've already done so many tests. How many more tests do we need? This is ridiculous!'

I had to admit, it did seem strange. Why was it necessary to repeat bloods again?

Dev stirred. 'Mum, just leave it. She's only doing her job. I don't mind, honestly.'

'I'm sorry about this,' I said. 'And I'm sorry you're in hospital over Diwali.'

'I'm alright,' he croaked. 'It is what it is. Got a gig soon,' he breathed. 'So I want this over and done with.'

I was taken aback. 'A gig, did you say? Are you a singer or something?'

'Recording artist. I write all my own material . . .'

'That is very cool,' I said.

Manisha was listening to our conversation.

'I'm going to be big. You wait and see.' Dev stared down at the mattress. 'Then I'm getting out of Levinstone.'

'My boy is talented,' whispered Manisha from the corner. 'He needs to be in rehearsals. Not stuck in hospital. I did not think we would be here during the Diwali festival.'

'We've still got another two days. You could be home in time for it. Maybe you can write some songs while you're in here. Don't forget where you come from when you're rich and famous.'

Dev groaned.

With everything done, I walked off heavy-footed down the corridor. To my relief, I caught sight of Nikolaus and admired his slender shoulders. He had his back turned. I imagined it was him in my bed last night, after the club.

'You off, then?' I said, beaming. I wanted to bring my face closer to his, just to inhale him.

He turned and smiled.

'I'm Nina,' I said, drawing closer, my skin prickling with heat.

'Pleased to meet you, Nina,' said Nikolaus, as if practising my name. I hoped that spoke of mutual interest.

We stood awkwardly for a second, unsure where to look.

'Is that an accent you have?'

He nodded. 'I'm German.'

'I guess the name gives it away.' I laughed nervously. *Stupid. Stupid.*

His eyes ran over my face.

I blushed, moving to the nurse's station as Nikolaus disappeared around the corner.

Checking the screen of my computer, I punched in a request for a doctor to see Dev. But waiting times had not changed.

By now it was getting too much; I needed air. I popped out of the ward for the canteen to pick up a soft drink, something sweet with vitamin C to keep me hydrated. I passed the phlebotomy department on the lower-ground floor and saw Arvin and Liam emerge from the entrance.

'Hi,' I said, 'how are you both?'

They feigned a smile and nodded, glancing at one another.

'Everything okay? I haven't seen either of you in ages.'

'As well as can be expected,' said Liam sulkily. His floppy blond hair and chubby cheeks made him appear extra spoilt.

'Not happy about what's going on. Richard pushing through unnecessary changes.' Arvin sucked in a long breath, sticking his belly out. He was like a newly appointed headteacher, placing his arms on his hips, thick fingers pinching his kidneys. 'Can't exactly compete when an external company is taking work, can we? Meanwhile, we're left with urgent turnaround tests, running around like headless chickens to try and meet targets.'

'You're talking about MediCentral?' I said.

'Who else?' said Liam. 'Today, routine and gold standard; tomorrow, all blood testing. Next time you see us, we might not have jobs.' Liam kicked at something imaginary on the floor. 'Might have to retrain and do something else.'

'I hear your frustration,' I said, 'but outsourcing is just to speed things up. With a rise in admissions, they won't reduce headcount. You're still very much needed.' But who was I kidding? Anything went. The management were under pressure and cost reductions usually meant one thing.

'This is just the start. I bet Richard has bigger plans,' said Arvin. 'You wait and see; it'll roll out further.'

I watched them walk off down the corridor.

'Stay positive!' I called.

Neither of them turned.

I rushed back to the ward, grateful to have had a few minutes to myself. Within seconds, Barry appeared at the door, his face weary, crashing me back down to earth. He waved at me through the glass as I stood at the nurse's station. Preeti passed, pressing the green buzzer to allow him to enter.

He trundled towards me like he was delivering bad news. It was all I needed, yet more doom and gloom.

'Just wanted a word before we bring him in,' Barry said. 'How are you?' His face was screwed tight and serious. 'Holding up okay, with everything going on?'

I walked towards him. His skin was blotchy, open pores. There were grey shadows beneath his eyes, and his shirt collar was sweat-stained.

'I will not lie. It's less than ideal. We're already overrun so we must prioritise better. Presumably you know about the raid. Heard how terrible it was?'

'I do, I do, but that's not why I'm here.'

Barry walked further into the ward.

'Tonight, the nurses are flat-out, the beds are full,' I said, walking alongside him. I heard coughing in the distance, a toilet flush. 'In here.'

I ushered Barry into the side office and we sat down in blue plastic chairs, opposite one another.

'It's about Leroy,' he said. 'He'll need to be kept apart from the others . . . ideally in a private room, his treatment prioritised because he has valuable information. If you could keep a close eye on him, I'd be ever so grateful.'

'I'm sorry?' I almost choked on my words.

'I appreciate there's been an incident,' he said, 'but we're operating in difficult circumstances. The sooner we see to him, the sooner he'll be out of here.'

I wanted to tell him I really didn't care. Those thugs were causing trouble, and Leroy was one of them. Why should I prioritise him? Was he at the raid? If so, he'd brought his stabbing on himself. I'd do my job, of course, but requesting special treatment and empathy and compassion to go along with it was asking a bit too much.

'I'm not in favour of them being given special treatment or private rooms,' I said. 'There are beds now occupied that should be given to more deserving patients.'

Barry shrugged. He stood, moving to the water cooler, and dispensed water into a cup. He took a sip, leaning on the windowsill. A flock of pigeons swooped past as he stared out of the window.

'Leroy is a grown man of twenty, trying to make something of himself,' he said. 'He got caught up with the wrong crowd because he was vulnerable. Are we saying he doesn't deserve to be treated equally?'

'Of course, he deserves *treatment*. I wouldn't be a nurse if I didn't think he did. But there are others out there waiting *ages* . . . It's difficult to reconcile prioritisation, is all I'm saying.'

Barry sniffed. 'Indiscriminate care, that's what free NHS healthcare is all about, isn't it?'

'I know my nursing code,' I said sarcastically. But I noted it was twice, now, that someone had questioned my comprehension of it.

'Leroy is a fine young man. You should hear how beautifully he speaks. I don't know, just as you don't know, how he ever ended up like this.'

'And I've got a wannabe popstar out there. But there's a big difference between them. Let's not get into a moral debate. Of course, we'll do whatever we can with limited space.'

Barry moved closer, staring into my eyes. 'We're closing

in on some of the key players responsible for terrorising the area. It won't be long, but we can't rush it.'

I clenched my toes, feeling the edge of the seat cutting into the back of my knees.

'Let's get him up on his feet as soon as we can.' Barry smiled cheerfully.

He threw his cup into the waste-paper basket.

'I'll have a police officer parked here. You'll be perfectly safe.'

# 7

Thirty minutes passed before the buzzer in the ward went off. I heard the fizz and crackle of a police radio, and an elderly porter wheeled Leroy into the private room. It all happened so fast I could barely keep up.

The private room was nice and clean. It had a sofa, TV, a view of the hospital green. Two police officers accompanied Leroy and helped the porter move him to the bed. I didn't offer to help. There were enough of them.

Leroy was flat on his back, breathing hard and fast. His way of coping with pain. Grinding his teeth, his nostrils flared. A patch of dry blood stained his neck, red splashes around his collar, one arm over his stomach. On his cheek was a large gash that looked like a tick. His skin was shiny where they'd applied antiseptic.

The porter wheeled the trolley out and the two police officers sat down.

He was just a kid, that much was clear. No matter how much Leroy tried to act like a grown man, he was incredibly juvenile. His face was boyish, borderline smug. Had he not been stabbed, tinselled in jewellery as he was, his wormy box braids beaded at the end, he could have been mistaken for having just returned from a beach holiday in St Lucia.

Barry hovered outside and nodded to me.

I tried to stay focused, blocking out everything. 'My name is Nina. I'll try to get you comfortable,' I mumbled.

He wore gold hooped earrings, a gold chain with a diamond cross. On his wrist, a chunky gold bracelet, thick like rope.

'You must be in a lot of pain,' I said, lowering his blanket, not thinking too much about it. I hitched up the side of his gown and he flinched.

'Fucking obvious, isn't it. You need to be careful, yeah? I'm not like the others. I need proper treatment.'

'Proper or *special*? Just so that I'm clear.' I carried out obs through gritted teeth.

One of the police officers cleared his throat.

From the corner of my eye, I saw Barry scrolling through his phone.

Leroy kissed his teeth like he'd rather not be here, as if *this*, all my medical attention, was a nuisance and interfered with his plans. I'd seen aggression like this before, normally drug-fuelled or relating to alcohol. Common, I found, with these sorts of people.

'Just hurry up,' he said.

I stared at my hands as they moved, the melanin in my skin the same as his. I'm half black, I thought, and yet, thankfully, nothing like him. 'I'm moving as quickly as I can. Just a few more minutes. I want to check your dressing.' How different we were, purely down to individual efforts. This man before me was behaving like a stereotype. He'd have no one to blame but himself if society labelled him.

A police officer rearranged himself in his seat.

I could see from the way his eyes bulged, Leroy was vexed. Maybe it was the weed, skunk, cocaine, whatever he was high on, that interfered with his ability to show kindness.

'Your quick ain't quick enough,' he spat.

‘Try not to talk. It’s unhelpful.’

He cut me a look, not expecting me to talk back.

‘It strains the abdomen,’ I said.

‘They fucking stabbed me!’ he said, his eyes piercing. He shuffled to lower himself. ‘They’re gonna pay. Like fuck, they’re gonna pay. I ain’t staying in here. No fucking way.’

I confess I wanted nothing more than for him to leave. To go get himself killed if that was what he wanted. I recorded his temperature, blood pressure, pulse. And, as per the notes, I’d need to draw blood for a routine examination. I caught a whiff of Leroy’s aftershave, musky with vanilla notes, the warm metal stench of blood as it oozed through his dressing. He stared at me as I pressed a gloved finger against the adhesive. My only priority that night was to make sure he did not soil the white blanket.

‘Oi, nurse. Look at me.’

I ignored him, moving back and forth from the metal trolley, laying out cotton and fresh dressings.

‘Have I seen you somewhere?’ he asked. ‘Cos I feel like I have.’

My stomach turned. ‘I doubt it,’ I said, but I felt it too. Something between us was strange and . . . familiar.

He raised his arm, and that was when I saw his wrist, a barbed-wire tattoo etched all around it.

I froze.

‘What’s wrong with you?’

My body trembled, the room around me blurred.

‘Why the fuck d’you keep staring at me like that?’

I moved my hands quickly, tugging at the corner of his dressing. I felt like ripping it off, slicing a blade through his stitches.

'Your dressing . . . it's soaked right through. I–I need to change it,' I said. But all I wanted was to get as far away from him as possible.

Leroy's head fell back onto the pillow. 'For fuck's sake. Hurry up.'

I moved to the corner, grabbing a pack of thicker dressings, scissors, tape, plastic to slide underneath him to protect the mattress. A cap lay on the chair next to his bed with the initials SK.

Caught between fear that he might recognise me and anger given his involvement in a violent crime, I felt my stomach burn. For a second, I thought I might wet myself. I tried to block negative thoughts, keeping myself occupied. I had to remind myself that I was duty-bound to remain indiscriminate. But I couldn't stand the thought of it. I was nursing a criminal, one I'd just witnessed at the raid, and so close to a man who had been stabbed. My stomach clenched. I thought of that man lying on the pavement and it made me sick – sick to the pit of my stomach. I was nursing *this* man when every instinct in my body told me to leave him to suffer.

I lowered my eyes, hoping he didn't clock it was me back there on the bus. I popped my head out of the room, calling out to Preeti for help.

She rushed in; the two of us went to work. She removed dressings from their wrapper, handing them to me. I pressed them down onto his stomach. Having cleaned him up, we left him in the recovery position.

'Everything alright here?' Barry approached me in the corridor.

'Need to talk to you now,' I said, breathless.

We hurried into the side room and I closed the door. The words hurtled out of my mouth before I could stop them. 'It's *him*. It's Leroy. He's part of the gang responsible for the rush outside Screaming Motors. I saw them – I saw *him*. He stabbed someone. I'm sure of it.'

'Nina . . .'

'I'm telling you it's *him*. You need to arrest him, Barry.'

He sighed. 'We're taking the event very seriously. He has some involvement, yes, but it's not what it seems. We've made several arrests and we're beginning an investigation.'

'So, you admit he was there when that man was stabbed?'

'I didn't say that.'

I stared at Barry, dumbfounded, then grabbed my phone. 'I have a video. I have Leroy filmed—'

I fumbled for my phone, thumbing through videos.

'We've received a lot of recordings and we're ploughing through them all. Look, Nina . . . I'm afraid I can't go into any of the details.'

It struck me as an odd thing to say.

'What the hell does that mean? I'm treating him when I *know* he's guilty.'

'If you'd rather switch nurses . . .'

I stared at Barry.

'. . . if it's proving difficult, I mean.'

'What *nurses*? There are no other nurses!' I said.

'Nina. I'm sorry.' Barry sat down. 'It's important you stay focused and, dare I say it, professional.'

I threw my head back and laughed. 'This is ridiculous. Do you know that? You're protecting a criminal.' I turned to leave, a part of me unsurprised by Barry's reaction – the sheer audacity of it.

He called after me. 'Wait! Nina—'

But by now I was walking fast down the corridor.

'Where are you going? We haven't finished!'

'To see my other patients,' I called.

He ran after me, grabbing my arm. 'Hang on! Leroy is priority – I did say.'

I shook him off, passing Dev, Colin, Marg, walking faster towards the kitchen. I needed water, something to cool me down.

A doctor dashed past me, tall, handsome and broad, his face the kind that appeared certain to achieve success if you saw it in a high-school photo. 'Nurse! I don't suppose you know where Leroy is – the stab-wound victim? Received an urgent call. Got here as quickly as I could.'

I pointed to the room in the corner and he dashed off. He had got here in ten minutes – a record given the backlog. Dev had been left waiting for God knows how long, but now, a doctor magically appeared to lavish Leroy with undue attention.

I craned my neck, hoping to avoid Manisha. I'd never be able to explain this.

Barry followed the doctor and I trailed behind, standing in the doorway as Barry entered. He moved closer to the doctor, whispering to him, laughing, joking, like they were the best of friends.

But Leroy was a criminal. I knew what I'd seen. And then there was Dev, a good Indian boy, struggling with no firm diagnosis, just a flimsy hypothesis.

Something inside me changed as if the dials of a safe had been turned. I washed my face and made my way to the medical supplies room, standing, staring at the door to the controlled drugs cabinet. I glanced down at the key in my hand.

That morning, after my shift, when Dev's bloods and samples came back normal and he was given a slot for his operation after waiting six hours, I found myself walking along the street in a stunned state. I was aware only of the tablets rattling around in my bag, firmly tucked under my arm. I had crossed a line by stealing morphine, but believed I had it in me to restrain myself from swallowing the tablets.

I walked as fast as I could, constantly looking behind me in case I was being followed.

There was an eeriness in the air, as if I was walking through a moment after a terrible event, the imprint, the muscle memory of it, hanging over me like a spider web.

Moving towards my flat, shoes squelching in the rain – oblivious to my clothes, soaking wet against my skin – I glanced up. There was a poster pinned to a tree, soggy, corners curling, and emblazoned with bold copy:

*Robbery and stabbing. Outside Screaming Motors. 26th October 2022 at 5 p.m. Did you see or hear anything? Call the number below with any information. £5,000 offered to anyone with key details leading to an arrest.*

I immediately recognised the man in the photo, grinning, arms crossed. His short, stout body . . . standing in front of the Samosa Hut.

*Balraj.*

# 8

That evening, I arrived at work a little early. I couldn't stop thinking about Balraj. How such a kind and considerate man could fall victim to such a cruel and callous crime. I was intent on locating the ward he'd been admitted to, and found him in the Lighthouse Tower, Newgate Hospital's trauma unit. I remembered his words: *Any problem, you come and see me. Balraj is here for you.*

I just couldn't believe it.

I stood beside his bed, noting the rise and fall of his chest amid the beep-beep-beep of the heart monitor. A tube trailed out of his nose and mouth. The air escaped his lips making a faint gurgling sound. I glanced at his face, his arms stickered with dressings over gashes and bruises, a dressing patched over his left eye. Every now and again, his right eye flickered.

Seated beside him was Sheela, rocking back and forth, dabbing her cheeks with the scraggly ends of her shawl. 'I told him so many times to be careful,' she said. 'He was not supposed to be there at that time. He knew how dangerous it was.'

Balraj's eyebrow twitched, and I wondered whether he could hear the two of us talking. I scanned his outline, saw his fingers move. After a few minutes, his right eye opened, and he stared up at the ceiling.

'Balraj?' I leaned closer.

Sheela shot up. 'You are awake, my love?'

'I am . . . awake,' he rasped. 'It is not so easy to sleep . . . hearing you both going on and on . . .'

Sheela and I glanced at one another and laughed, her eyes bright with tears.

'I'm so sorry.' I shook my head, feeling an intense anger rise from the pit of my stomach. 'I feel so *helpless*.'

'It is not your fault,' Sheela said. 'Someone bad is responsible. Balraj has done much good for this community and is harmless. I cannot understand why this happened – why he would be a target.'

'He just got in the way, that's all,' I said. 'But the person responsible won't get away with it.' I saw Leroy so clearly in my mind.

Balraj swallowed; his Adam's apple bobbed and slipped.

'Maybe it is not one person,' said Sheela. 'There were almost thirty young men.'

'But only one held the knife,' I said.

I placed my hand on Balraj's hand, feeling the touch of his leathery skin.

'I cannot allow myself . . . to be angry,' croaked Balraj.

'Well, we are all here praying for you to get better,' warbled Sheela. She placed a hand to her mouth to cover her quivering lip.

I turned to Sheela. 'What are the police doing about this? Did you speak to them? Should I?'

'What can they do? They do not know who is responsible. Too many people involved. They will wait for Balraj to feel stronger,' she said. 'Then they will start their questions all over again.'

'CCTV? I could provide a statement – I was there. I have a video . . . it is a little grainy, but CCTV might be better.'

'Masks,' strained Balraj. 'They had masks.'

'The police checked,' said Sheela.

I clenched my jaw. 'They planned this well,' I said.

'There are many videos,' said Sheela, downcast. 'The police said it is not enough.'

I shook my head, wanting to change the subject.

'I brought you some flowers,' I said quickly. I pulled them out of a bag beside my knee, holding them upright. I'd tied them with a red ribbon. Pink dahlias, stolen from the flower box outside number eighty-four. Sheela lifted the bunch suspiciously. She left the room in search of a vase.

'We're going to get whoever did this, I promise.' I reached out to grasp Balraj's hand. It broke me to see a tear trickling from the corner of his eye. I gripped his hand more tightly.

'It is my bad karma . . . returning to punish me.'

'Don't be ridiculous. How can any of this be your fault?'

He shook his head. '"He who wields the knife does not hold it alone when it plunges . . ." That is what Pastor Otis said . . . "We are all cloaked in collective failure."' He began coughing, spluttering.

I bolted forward. 'Go easy, Balraj. You're still very weak.'

'I remember his words more clearly than my own . . .'

'Otis is a good man,' I said, 'he means well. But he's not thinking straight. Those criminals must be held accountable. They need locking up in jail.'

I felt a fire rising inside me as I recalled the community meeting, how unsatisfactory and inconclusive it was.

Sheela returned, her eyes puffy, wiping her nose with a tissue.

'I had better go and start my shift,' I said. It hurt to stay there any longer. 'I'll come back soon, I promise. Just let me know if you need help with anything.'

Sheela nodded.

Balraj gently closed his eyes.

On my way out, I went to search for the nurse in charge. Her name was Felicity Mayhew, a get-it-done kind of nurse, uninterested in politics or hospital gossip. The kind I liked who focused only on her patients. She'd graduated from the same college as I did almost ten years ago, but since then, we'd hardly spoken.

'Good to see you, Nina. It's bad news, I'm afraid. The odds are stacked against him.' Felicity glanced down, unable to meet my eye. 'He's sustained a stab wound to the right flank producing immediate paralysis in both legs. Recovery is possible, but chances are slim. If mobility does return, it'll be slow in coming.'

I shook my head, the weight of the tragedy too heavy to bear.

'I wish I could say it's a one-off,' she said, 'but incidents like this are becoming all too common.' She sighed. 'It's what it's like around here. A part of me thinks we need to grow to accept it.'

'But you'll make sure he gets proper care, won't you? No matter how bad the shortages.'

Felicity nodded. 'I'll do my best. But you know how it is. Priorities shift and change all the time. Resources are limited.'

I walked through the stale corridor leading to Florence Nightingale, overcome by a sense of virtue and moral justice. It was not right; *nothing* about this situation was right. More than anything else in the world, I wanted to teach Leroy Sanchez a lesson. The police had failed to intervene to protect this town – my home, and its good people. I knew that Leroy was responsible for what happened. I knew what I'd seen – him running away. Why would he do that if he was innocent?

I had just started my shift. But before I could settle in, the buzzer in Leroy's room went off – a continual buzz, then a series of pulses. The policeman snoozing in a chair outside Leroy's room jolted as I dashed past him. I gritted my teeth, entering the private room with every ounce of flesh in my body, resistant. The skin along my arms felt thick and numb.

'What do you want?' I asked, my voice heavy as I towered over Leroy. He lay on his side, face tilted towards me. His eyes were bright and round, piercing my skin like a needle.

'Nurse Nina,' he said as if we enjoyed a personal relationship, as if my whole existence revolved around his.

I switched on the light, the sudden brightness startling him. He cowered, covering his eyes. 'You need to give me notice when you do that!' he cried. 'I'm still weak, y' know!'

For a second, I imagined slicing the fingers off his dry, calloused hands.

I kept thinking, *No one knows how exhausted I am, how I'm now having to nurse a criminal.*

Leroy groaned. 'There's something wrong with me. I think I'm . . . leaking.'

I rolled my eyes; it was all I needed.

'Leaking, where?' I didn't want to touch him if I could at all help it.

'Something is torn. I can feel it.'

His notes confirmed he'd been seen by Sandra an hour before I'd started my shift, given a painkiller and then left to doze off in a blissful sleep. Stupid man must have moved about, causing his own rupture.

I grabbed a fresh pair of gloves, then lowered his blanket, lifting his arm crookedly into the air. I asked him to roll onto his side so I could pull up his gown. His dressing was soiled in blood, creamy pus running down his side like melted butter.

'When did this happen?' I asked, pursing my lips. The dressing needed a change, but by God, I couldn't be bothered to do it.

'I don't know. You're the nurse, you work it out.'

'Did you try to get out of bed – only to strain yourself?'

Leroy was silent. I imagined he did move. I knew if it was really bad, I'd have to call the doctor.

'All I did was bend a bit to charge my phone.'

I peeled off the edge of the plaster and he squirmed. Thankfully, the stitches were intact. Just a bit of pus and blood leaking from the side, that was all it was. It was best to take a swab.

I carried out the usual obs and began to change his dressing, pleasured by the thought that, at least now, he knew what it felt like to be in pain. He'd been stabbed himself, and he deserved it.

I moved sluggishly, retrieving cotton wool, surgical tape,

a roll of plasters. I helped ease Leroy into a comfortable position, laying him on his side, slowly peeling off his bandage. 'Sorry, it's stuck to your skin.' I wanted to rip it off so badly and to hear him sing.

His body stiffened.

I took a swab of the pus to send to the lab, noting there was no spreading redness, no sign of infection, and mopped up the mess with cotton wool. I replaced the covering with a fresh one. He clenched his jaw, and it dawned on me just how much he hurt. He put on a good show, but I'd seen over the years how pain could reduce a grown man to tears.

I replaced his gown, tucking him back into his blanket. 'There. You're fine now. Probably just need to sleep it off.'

I cleared up the dirty dressings, ripping the gloves off to thoroughly wash my hands.

'Sleep, through this?' he called as my back turned.

'Sure. After an injection, that is.' The soap on my hands was warm and slippery.

I turned, enjoying the sight of the terror in his eyes, that sight of sheer helplessness and surrender to the power I commanded now.

'It's been more than three hours since your last painkiller,' I said. 'I'd recommend you take it.'

He glared at me, uncertain whether there was something he'd missed.

'Can't I just have a tablet?'

'An injection's quicker.'

He swallowed.

I wiped my hands on a paper towel and tossed it into the bin.

'I don't want any needles. I don't consent,' he whispered. 'Why can't you do it in the cannula?'

'I'll use that for IV fluids and antibiotics if you need it. Let's see what the swab results say.'

I took a step forward and he recoiled, as if the prospect of a needle was more terrifying than jail.

I laughed. 'Don't tell me you're afraid of needles.' I got myself a fresh pair of gloves.

'Fuck off!' he said. 'Don't make fun of me.'

His body trembled, and inside, I was roaring.

'You'll feel better,' I said. 'Try to relax. Enjoy it.'

'Seriously, go fuck yourself!' He flinched under the blanket.

'Come along now . . . be a big boy about it.'

He jerked harder. 'Well, go on then, psycho. Get it over with!'

Outside I thought I heard Dev, but I couldn't be sure.

I snapped open a mini glass ampoule of fentanyl, inserting the needle into the liquid. I felt the low pressure inside the syringe as the plunger pulled back.

'I'll inject this into your vein, which will be the quickest way for you to experience relief. It works almost straight away but might make you feel . . . drowsy.'

God, I was tired.

Leroy bit his lip so hard it appeared to be turning blue. His breaths were quick and shallow.

I swept a ball of cotton wool into the crease of his elbow and held the needle at ninety degrees, pressing the sharp tip of it directly onto his skin.

He squeezed his eyes closed; I thought I heard him squeal.

I held the needle there for a few seconds longer to make him really *feel* it.

I laughed under my breath, finally plunging the needle into his arm. Relishing the prick as it pierced into flesh, I plunged the liquid down through the syringe, delighting in the whooshing sound.

'Why would anyone want to stab you?' I asked as I slid the needle out.

His shoulders fell and he released a long exhale. He licked his lips to speak. 'People don't want you to do anything on their parts. But you do what you can to protect yourself . . . and others.'

'What do you mean?'

'Does it matter? Why the fuck do you care?'

Leroy seemed aware of how his voice had changed.

'Because I live here, that's why. I don't want your sort causing trouble around here. Presumably you heard about that poor Sikh man who got stabbed. You must have heard – and *seen* what happened.'

He fell silent. 'Best you don't go running your mouth if you don't know anything, yeah? That video had nothing to do with me. I got caught up in it, and then . . . I couldn't get out.'

He'd obviously been told about the videos.

'I see.'

I pressed a plaster down over his skin. He fell back onto the pillow as if the sheer effort of watching me work had taken everything out of him. He stared up at the ceiling, at something in the distance. Perhaps he was thinking about his life, his circumstances. The clarity and precision of the needle.

I gathered my things, popping the cotton swabs, plastic

wrappings, the used syringe into the appropriate bins. I replaced his blanket, despising him with every cell in my body. So consumed was I with hatred, my body and mind no longer felt connected. I tore off my gloves and washed my hands. I switched off the light and was about to walk out the door, but unable to keep his mouth shut, Leroy called out to me once more.

'What is it?' I mumbled in the dark.

'I know who you are.'

I stopped dead in my tracks.

'It was you, wasn't it? Staring at me from the bus.'

I bit the inside of my cheek, feeling the saliva pool inside my mouth.

'It wasn't supposed to happen. Not like that. Nobody was supposed to get hurt.'

I couldn't move. I felt a fire burning inside me, overcome by the urge to press a pillow onto his face, so that I would never, ever have to deal with him again.

'But they did get hurt. A man, much loved in the community, was maimed,' I said.

'You don't understand. You don't know what's going on. What you saw that night is not what happened.'

My body stiffened.

'Go to sleep, Leroy. I'd rather you didn't strain your wound. Enough taxpayers' money is being spent on taking care of you.'

I closed the door behind me as the policeman outside straightened in his chair.

'Is everything alright?' he asked.

'Everything is just perfect,' I said.

# 9

Wearily, I moved about the ward as thoughts of exacting justice bubbled and stirred. I wondered how much more of this I could take. I was thinking of the morphine I'd stolen, how I could do with it now. I snapped back into action when I went to check on Dev. Manisha bolted out of her chair as I approached his bed.

'He's had an operation but he's still suffering.' Her body shook. She bit the skin around her nails. She looked terrible, like a feral animal, hair loose and wild, eyes red and bulging.

'I'm sorry to hear that,' I said.

I checked over Dev's notes written by an agency nurse standing in to cover the previous day.

The notes confirmed that Dev had been to theatre earlier, at 1 p.m., wheeled back into Florence Nightingale to recover at 5 p.m. He'd been prescribed two tablets of morphine to take orally, 10mg each, to help ease his pain. He'd had the usual obs, his temperature logged – still too high at 38°C. Another FBC to check for signs of post-op infection. All clear. No indication in the notes of what might be required next.

'I can't understand what it could be. He should be feeling better by now. Especially since we've carried out so many tests and found nothing.' I moved closer to Dev and saw how frail he was, curled up in a foetal position, unable to even glance up. 'I'll call the doctor.'

Manisha moved to the window, her gaze frantically darting about the blue curtains.

'Did he take the morphine prescribed?' I asked. I bit my lip.

Manisha shook her head. 'He doesn't need it,' she said, her voice clipped. 'I will not allow it.'

'Where are the tablets?'

She was silent, thinking. I glanced at the bin, certain the tablets were in there. I wanted to fish them out so badly.

'There's no point giving him tablets until we know why his health is not improving after the operation,' she said. 'But of course, no doctor is available to see my son. I don't know how much more of this I can take.'

I reread the notes, trying to stay focused. 'If there was any cause for concern, they would have told you by now.'

'Well, they *didn't*!' She sat down. 'This space is horrible. We've heard coughing, spluttering, all afternoon. The smell of the food is enough to make anyone want to vomit.'

I held on to my stomach, aware of just how hungry I was. I would gladly eat something now. Shepherd's pie. Cauliflower cheese. Whatever they had left over in the kitchen.

'I'm afraid there's nowhere else he can go,' I said. I was way out of my depth. We had done everything right. Carried out all manner of tests in A&E, ASU – pre- and post-op. But each one turned out to be negative. I couldn't understand it.

I called for a doctor several times. Eventually, Dr Milburn wandered in, an overgrown child in a short, stubby body. He peered down at Dev, scraping his teeth against his bottom lip as he concentrated.

'So let us be clear . . .' he said, swiping a hand over his fringe that hung over his brow like a curtain.

'Since Dev's arrival, we've carried out all the necessary tests. But . . . we've found nothing.'

Manisha leaned forward and held Dev's hand.

'Even with an appendectomy, the patient's pain persists.'

'Isn't that obvious?' said Manisha. 'What is it that we *do* moving forward?' She sat with her back bent, the cuffs of her jumper pulled over her hands. She couldn't stop fidgeting.

'Mmm . . .' Dr Milburn skimmed the notes. 'It *is* worrying. We could do a CT scan to see if there's anything that needs attention post-op. This will give us a detailed picture of his organs, from his lower chest to his pelvis. It will allow us to effectively diagnose and assess possible treatment. But I must warn you, it might take a while. It's busy in the hospital tonight.'

Manisha squeezed her eyes closed.

'It's also possible – and highly probable – that this may just clear up on its own. We ought to give it more time before considering referral. A CT scan for now is sufficient. We'll just need to give Dev a little contrast solution to drink so that the imaging is clearer. It's perfectly safe.'

Manisha bolted up. 'What?' Her eyes were wide, menacing. 'He is not drinking any such thing.'

'Actually, I don't mind that,' said Dev. 'I'm fed up with being prodded . . . so if it helps . . .'

'No! Nothing here is to be trusted. Why can't you do it without the solution?'

'We can. If you prefer,' said Dr Milburn.

'It would make the scan more accurate,' I said. 'There's really nothing to worry about.'

'I said no, thank you. How much more do you expect my son to take?' The exasperation in Manisha's voice was so pronounced, she sounded hoarse. 'We've been here for *two days* and it's Diwali in a few hours. We'll even have a new prime minister! But still, we are no wiser as to what's going on.'

'I'm sorry—' I said, feeling utterly helpless.

'I know you are,' Manisha cut in. 'But your sorry doesn't help us move forward, does it?'

If I was being honest, a part of me was detaching.

'Mum,' said Dev, 'calm down, okay?' He pulled the blanket to his neck, his hands shaking from the sheer effort of it.

I approached. 'Try and relax.'

Dev nodded, his eyes searching mine, silently pleading for help.

I saw a rash breaking over Dev's cheeks, so I washed my hands and pulled on a pair of gloves to examine it.

'I wish they would stop,' whispered Dev as I drew my face closer to his.

I heard Manisha arguing with Dr Milburn, begging him to do *something more*.

'We're doing everything we can,' I said, focusing only on the patient in front of me, just like I was trained to do. 'I'll get you some hydrocortisone cream for that rash and a Piriton tablet.'

'It's not that simple.' Dr Milburn, again. 'We've had many patients seeking treatment. If there was anything more to suggest, we surely would. But in all my years of experience, I can tell you that after an appendectomy is carried out, some pain is to be expected. If there's anything serious, a CT scan will detect it. But if you'd rather he did that without contrast solution, that's fine.'

Manisha fell back into her seat as if all energy had left her body, and now she was worn out by nobody listening. 'At first, I didn't believe all the rumours about this hospital,' she said. 'But now I see it's true. You people don't care about patients.'

Dr Milburn rolled his eyes. 'Please let's focus on your son.'

'How dare you patronise me!' spat Manisha. 'That is precisely what I *am* doing. I'm giving him the attention you people have no time for.'

I turned to face them, my ears ringing. I took a deep breath and caught a glimpse of Marg stirring. Colin was sitting up, reading the paper. Pretending not to listen.

'We should take this conversation outside,' I said. Both were being ridiculous, behaving like children.

In the corridor, Dr Milburn asked me whether he could have a word.

'Trust me when I say that I've seen cases like this a thousand times before.'

'I was going to recommend—'

'Don't succumb to the melodrama, Nina. We must remain impartial – objective,' he said, scribbling on Dev's medication chart. '*We* are the medical professionals, and that woman is a menace.' He scratched his head. 'CT scan. Minus the contrast. Plus, additional morphine – ten milligrams. A tablet every six hours as needed, but for no more than two days.' He handed me the chart, turning on his heels.

He waved as he walked off through the double doors. I stared down at the prescription in my hands, knowing Manisha would not want Dev to take morphine because she'd already declined that as well. I knew this new prescription ought to be kept. That I could administer the morphine and let Dev refuse it, but for some reason – *stupid, stupid* – I thought I'd delete all record of it. These tablets, I wanted for myself. With all the pressure I was under, I knew – instinctively – I was building up to the moment when I might need it. It was the only way I could see myself coping. One tablet, here and there, was harmless.

I folded the chart, slipping it neatly into my breast pocket. I had resolved to make a fresh chart, doctoring the information.

By now, Manisha was stomping around, speaking into her phone, loudly. She complained about how ridiculous the doctor was, how *disgraceful* the hospital service. I wanted to ask Manisha to please stop using her phone in the ward. To remind her that the signal interfered with life-saving equipment. But I was afraid of what she might do. I did not want to risk upsetting the other patients.

I returned to Dev's bed; he was lying flat on his back, his eyes closed. I stared down at him, this most peculiar case. Appendicitis was the diagnosis, but could that be all this was?

He opened his eyes. 'I need to ask you something.'

'What is it?'

'It's a bit private.'

'I see . . .' I strained my neck to make sure Manisha was still some distance away. I pulled the curtains fully closed around us. 'How can I help?'

'I've done some bad things . . .'

I was taken aback. 'Bad, like what?' He'd piqued my interest, now.

'It's a bit delicate.'

'Go on.'

'Do you think the prolonged use of . . . well, weed, could mess up my stomach? I've been racking my brains, trying to figure out what could be wrong with me. I think it's that, but I can't say – not in front of my mum.'

I was amused that Dev was not the good boy Manisha believed him to be. Weed? Was he serious? What else had he been taking?

'We ought to let the doctor know. It's probably not relevant but we should make note of it on your record.'

'Nah! Don't do that. Mum'll go ballistic. Brought me up good 'n' proper. Look at me. Good Indian boy, and ever so handsome.'

He coughed into his hand as he struggled to laugh.

'How much have you been smoking, exactly?'

'A lot. I have suppliers, see. It's a bit of a side business. Funds my music. Because I sell, I need to do a bit of . . . product testing.'

I felt disappointed to hear this. I had grown fond of Dev and thought so much better of him. But his disclosure was confidential. His dealing had nothing to do with his clinical care. I placed my hand on his to provide reassurance. 'Your secret is safe with me. But you ought to tell the doctor about your consumption of weed. Also, just to remind you, you're a grown man . . . you don't need your mother's permission to make certain choices.'

He licked his lips and smiled. 'Mum's still getting used to that. You know how mothers are.'

But that was it: I didn't. I'd never known anything like a mother's presence. To me, it was nice, comforting – something I would have killed to have had growing up. Overbearing and militant was preferable to complete absence.

I turned to leave, but Dev called after me. 'I think he likes you,' he croaked.

I was taken aback.

'That porter. The one that brought me here. He likes you – if you're interested.'

My stomach flipped; my shoulders fell. 'You really think so?' Just the thought of Nikolaus made me feel warm.

Dev smiled. 'I know that look when a man likes a woman. I know . . . you like him, as well.'

I drew close, ruffling his hair. 'You are a funny one,' I said.

# 10

I walked to Levinstone Library, a grey and shabby building, the surrounding canal murky and littered with floating fags and crushed beer cans. I felt the first chill of winter through my flimsy coat. In the distance, a woman approached.

'I'm glad you called,' Farah said. 'It's funny because I knew you would.' She sat down next to me, a polystyrene cup in hand. The steam trailed in the breeze as cars whizzed by.

'Shall we go someplace else?' I asked. I'd wanted this meeting to be discreet. There was so much I needed to tell her about Leroy, and here felt risky. 'There's a McDonald's a few doors down.'

Farah nodded. Inside, she placed our order. Hers, a cheeseburger meal with strawberry milkshake. Mine, a chicken salad. When I turned, I realised how pretty Farah was. It was something I hadn't noticed before. Her eyes were clear like glass, reflecting intelligence and confidence.

We walked with our food towards an unoccupied alcove. I sat down, twisting the cap on my bottle of water, making myself feel comfortable.

'So, what's this about?' Farah unwrapped her burger and took a bite. Chomping, she covered her mouth with her hand. 'Not exactly halal. But *shhhh*! Don't tell anyone.' She laughed.

'I have some important evidence about a crime.'

'Oh?'

'A video of the attack against Balraj Singh. The one outside Screaming Motors.'

Farah dabbed her lips with a tissue. 'Can I see the video?' she said, covering her mouth again. Her eyes narrowed; a finger was smeared with ketchup.

I handed her my phone, watching as she licked her fingers. She pressed PLAY. Her eyes flickered, brows raised as sounds emanated from the phone's speakers. I found myself holding my breath. But to my surprise, she returned the phone after only a few seconds.

'I've received a few of these, I'm afraid. We've already run the story. Gang rivals, battling it out. An innocent local caught up in the moment. It's live on our website.'

I leaned in closer, unable to believe what she'd just said. I couldn't understand how she could be so dismissive of hard evidence. 'But I know who did it!'

'Go on.'

'I saw the young man involved – saw him with my own eyes. He is now a patient at Newgate. You need to investigate it.' The more I relayed the story, the more I grew certain of it.

'*Your* patient, did you say?' Farah placed her burger down, lifting her milkshake.

I shook my head. 'No, not mine, exactly, but on the ward. The police know he did it but are covering it up. That's the bit I don't understand.'

She stared at me. 'I'll need stronger evidence to substantiate what you're saying. Also, you should know, we have an agreement with the local police. We need to give them a heads-up before running a story that might undermine them.'

I leaned back in my chair. 'It's not just me. There will be others who saw him, too. I'm sure of it.'

'Who is he?' she asked.

'His name is Leroy Sanchez. Part of a gang but acts like the leader. He's under police protection while he's receiving treatment.'

She grabbed my phone, watching the video once more. 'I can't see his face. And it's all a bit . . . grainy.'

'He's wearing a balaclava.'

She sighed. 'I'm sorry. It's simply not strong enough.'

'But I know the man they attacked. I live in his flat!' I knew I was losing ground, clutching hard on a rope slipping and burning through my hands. I glanced down. 'He did a lot for me. I wouldn't be where I am now if it wasn't for his kindness.'

Farah pursed her lips. 'It's libellous to implicate a man in a crime without any firm evidence. Have you anything else?'

My mind was scrambling. 'Like what, exactly?'

'I mean, any dirt on Newgate. Park this story for now. What I'm interested in is anything you've got on what's going on since Richard's arrival.'

I scanned the restaurant to make sure no one there would recognise me. I had to tell her something to save myself from losing face. 'The new management is problematic,' I whispered.

'In what way?'

I told her what I knew: that there was a financial black hole that departments were now under pressure to fill. 'They've cut corners all over the place. We're struggling with staff shortages. Waiting times are criminal. On top of it all, nurses have suffered assaults from the influx of casualties caught up in gang activity. Mark my words, something terrible will happen . . .'

'Do you think someone like Richard is aware of the implications day to day?' she asked. She pulled out a notebook from her bag, flicking through the pages. 'Does he know that standards have slipped? I'm not sure if you're aware, but there's a lot of reported incidents concerning patient care. I've spoken to a few nurses. It seems they've all been told – *threatened* – to keep quiet.'

I felt a shiver run down my spine.

'It makes me mad, really it does, that sick people are not getting proper treatment. The public deserves to know what's going on.'

'All I know is that we're overstretched,' I said. 'When there's already a lack of government funding and a mismanagement of existing budgets, it's obvious that patient care will suffer. I suppose Richard's changes are intended to make things more efficient. Not everyone agrees with it, though. Truth be told, I don't either. It's unfair to blame care workers for slippages if the hospital is overwhelmed. That's too easy.'

I stared down at my food, my appetite lost.

'Maternity is the biggest problem, from what I hear,' Farah said. 'Three deaths, all mothers. Three unexplained – newborns. At my last count, ten unexplained fatalities across various parts of the hospital.'

My chest tightened. A wave of panic washed over me. I thought of Mercedes, whether she knew to what extent people were watching her. 'Are they blaming nurses?'

'People will eventually, because you are the faces of the NHS.'

'But that's unfair.'

'So, we need to gather evidence of wider organisational failings.' Farah toyed with her French fries. 'What caused the financial black hole, do you know?'

'No clue.'

'Can you find out? Without that, powerful institutions will always use the little people as scapegoats.'

I took a bite of lettuce; the leaves were tasteless. I didn't know how I was getting embroiled in all this when all I wanted was justice for Balraj.

'Would you be willing to keep an eye out?' Farah said. 'Maybe for something to prove the financial black hole and how it happened. We need to tell the story of the impact of bad management on care provision.'

I stared down, and after a while, I nodded. 'I'll try,' I said. For sure, I didn't want nurses blamed for all the good they did. That seemed bang out of order.

Farah smiled. 'Thank you, Nina. I can't tell you how good it is to have someone like you looking out for the rest of us.'

That early afternoon, after I showered and changed into a fresh sweatshirt and joggers, I pulled open the top drawer of my side cupboard. There were loose pens, bits of paper, a few of the morphine tablets I'd swiped from Newgate.

I stared at the strip of purple pills with 'RD 71' printed in the centre. I popped one out of the plastic bubble, holding it, a little moon, in the centre of my palm, delighting in how comforting it felt. I placed two tablets on the tip of my tongue, closed my eyes and swallowed.

My mind drifted as my body finally relaxed. I was overcome by a feeling of detachment, which I welcomed with open arms. A torrent of tiredness, regret, disappointment crashed over me. Strange shapes, colours, patterns floated across my eyelids.

I saw a scarf, trailing in the breeze. It turned into a ripple, a wave, a river rushing towards the sea. When I opened my eyes, still locked inside a dream, I was on a bus, on the upper deck. My feet lay anchored to the floor, my hands pressed flat onto the velvety seat cover. I recalled that triangle-shaped gap between a pair of joggers. Balraj's cheery face, up close, filled with terror.

And then there he was. Leroy. I banged on the window, screaming *Leave him alone! Someone help him! Please, someone help Balraj!* I wanted, so desperately, to rush down the stairs, to smash through the bus doors, to burst out onto the pavement. I saw a trickle of blood run onto the kerb. Grabbing my phone, I frantically dialled emergency services. I was begging, pleading for them to help him. When someone finally answered – a woman, her voice calm and polished, asking me what the nature of my emergency was – the call got disconnected.

I bolted upright in bed. I felt a drop of sweat run slowly down my neck.

After that, I couldn't sleep. I kept thinking about Balraj. Heard him laugh. Recalled a few of the conversations we'd had. I remembered a story he'd once told me about how he'd come up with the idea for the Samosa Hut. An ode to his mother who discovered she had a knack for making them. He'd said she started making them when at home, raising himself and his two brothers. Word caught on once a few people had tasted them. She prepared hundreds for the locals in her village to keep up with demand. But then, when I remembered how he'd served me a plate on my very first day, moving into his flat, I saw his blue scarf soaked in blood all over again.

I switched on the TV for a little sound. I played YouTube yoga videos to distract myself. I did some chores, folding clothes, ironing, wiping down the windows. I scrubbed the kitchen sink so hard a strand of steel wire became trapped inside my fingertip.

*Fucking moron, useless cow. Pick up the fluff from the carpet with your own bare hands.*

I stabbed and picked at my skin with a needle, prising out the bit of wire, watching how the blood bobbled and oozed all the way down to my wrist.

When I couldn't take it anymore, I threw on my coat. I needed to be in the only place where I knew I would find some peace. I made my way down Oldfield Lane, passing shops with barricaded windows, past the Carnival Pot restaurant, still open, that served its famous curried goat cooked with secret Jamaican spices.

I walked in a sedated daze, ambling in the cold and rain, until I saw the bar-and-circle sign for Levinstone Tube station.

Once on the Tube, I took a seat by the window. My chest grew tight as it always did. Because to everyone else making this journey, it might appear routine, travelling to work, to a bar or restaurant, then back home again to sleep. But to me, it meant so much more than that. This journey was deep, meaningful. Like a homecoming.

At Westminster, I got off the Tube, walked up the marble stairs, heading towards the Houses of Parliament. The crowds around me moved like thick treacle. I imagined politicians, ministers, important persons engaged in the formation of a new cabinet. Rishi Sunak was due to be our new prime minister. Everyone was discussing how he'd face unprecedented challenges. Here we were, hurtling into winter with high energy bills, long hospital waiting times, soaring inflation rates. I couldn't help but wonder how much he knew of the life led by most people propping up Great Britain.

I crossed my bag over my chest, the bulk of it pressed against my hip. I wondered whether a visit like this, today, just before Diwali, meant it was more auspicious. A strange calm washed over me as I walked towards Parliament Square, heading for the familiar tall red box just beside Big Ben.

Inhaling the stale stench of cigarettes, standing outside the usual realms of life and death, negotiating the fragility of people's existence, I found I was moving deeper inside myself.

Here, inside the comfort of a box-like existence, I at least knew where I was: on solid ground, with perhaps even a little certainty to rely on. I'd memorised the phone number by heart. Said it out loud repeatedly to myself. All these years, not once had it changed. That number said more about who I was and where I came from than my own birth certificate.

I was about to pick up the phone, imagining a voice on the other end of the line, a woman who might tell me what I'd always wanted to know: why I was abandoned as a baby and dumped inside a telephone box.

There was a knock on the window. As I looked up, I saw a man with a snarly face, a cigarette trailing from his lips. *Will you be long?* he mouthed. I offered him a nod, a downward glance. Grabbing a pen and blank card from my bag, I frantically began scribbling:

> *I'm appealing to anyone with information about my mum and dad. I was left here in a basket on 21 March 1995, found by a passer-by at 2 a.m. After that, I was handed over to social services and grew up in care. I just want to find my parents, or even just one of them – either my mum or dad – whoever is around. I suspect my mum is Indian and my dad is black. If anyone has any information, please call me on my mobile.*

I pinned the card to the wall, next to pink cards advertising Thai call girls. It was the same card I left each time I visited, usually three times a year, with, by now, no expectation of ever receiving a reply.

I stepped out of the phone box and into the cold, heading back to the Tube station for home.

# 11

That evening, as the morphine wore off, the crumpled edge of myself returned. In the staff toilets, I stared at my face, hardly recognising the woman I saw reflected in the mirror.

Leaning over the sink, I splashed cold water onto my eyes, head heavy in my hands. My mouth tasted of metal; the fug of morphine had left with it a strange, fragmented feeling. Drying my face with a paper towel, the texture rough against my skin, I straightened my scrubs and re-arranged my name tag.

I was not addicted. I'd only taken two tablets. Just something to help me cope. It wouldn't happen again – definitely not.

I felt a tightness in my chest. The air around me crackled; a high-pitched ringing pierced my ears. I wanted desperately to cry out, felt as if the concrete around me was crumbling. My scrubs felt stiff, my body drenched in pain. In and out, I fired quick breaths to calm myself down again.

Something worked, something was shifting. I did it all by myself, and without any morphine.

I needed to check up on Dev, so I walked into the corridor just as Barry trundled past, heading towards Leroy's room.

He whispered to the police officer parked by the door. The officer closed his book and left. Barry entered the room alone and the door quietly closed behind him.

Instinctively, I stood outside the room. In the warm, stuffy corridor, I heard the white noise of the PC monitor, the clink and groans of the radiators as water trickled through the channels. In the distance, the tip-tip-tip of water dripping from a tap. Through a gap in the curtains, I peered through the glass.

Barry was standing over the bed, a hand placed on Leroy's shoulder as Leroy lay on his side, his back bent, knees tucked. Barry was saying something to him – I couldn't make out what. But Leroy was listening attentively as he gazed at the floor.

After a few minutes, Barry took a step back and sat down on the visitor's chair. I saw the back of his fat head, heard him crack his neck. He crossed his legs, stretching his arms over his head like he didn't have a care in the world.

I checked the side of me, to be sure no one was about. I pressed my ear closer to the glass, feeling it warm against the helix.

Inside, the two men were still talking. Their voices, muffled; their words, just about audible: 'It's just a close call, that's all . . . We need not draw attention to it. We need to be careful,' said Barry.

'Yeah, well how the fuck was I to know everyone would be filming,' said Leroy.

'You can understand how this looks.' Barry sighed. 'The worst thing that can happen is that we press charges.'

Leroy stirred and Barry stood up, his back obscuring the bed. I strained harder still to listen, but could only hear snatches of their conversation.

'I tried to get there as fast as I could, yeah? You were supposed to protect me but left me dangling like a dickhead.'

Barry shook his head. 'I'm there for you, not the rest of them. But why so many?'

'What was I supposed to do?' said Leroy. 'Easy for you to say – you and the rest of them. Coppers protected by their uniform.'

Barry sighed. 'You knew exactly what you were getting into.'

At the time, I didn't know what all this meant. It sounded to me like the police were protecting gang members. I remembered what Barry had said: *We're closing in on some of the key players . . . It won't be long.* This was altogether different.

My head was spinning because although we'd had our differences and he could be annoying, I'd always had Barry down as being one of the few good men left standing in the community. He was a straight copper in an increasingly crooked area. So, what was most disappointing in all this was that it confirmed everyone's natural suspicions about the police – that they always looked for the easy way out, even if that meant crossing a line to get the job done. I had no doubt that maybe Leroy was useful. But instead of locking up criminals, here they were, cutting shady deals. I wondered what people would say if a conversation like this ever got out. To think Barry was working with the man responsible for stabbing Balraj – and in the very hospital where Balraj lay crippled.

Before I could stop myself, I barged into the room. The two men flinched as I stood there, breathless.

'Hope I'm not breaking up the party,' I said.

'You could knock,' spat Leroy. 'Didn't your mother teach you any manners?'

I clenched my jaw, determined not to let him crawl under my skin, but his talk of my mother cut particularly deep.

I moved to the foot of his bed, lifting the clipboard to check his notes. He was recovering well. Stitches holding up. Wound healing. Nothing unusual detected in his swab results. *How nice for him.*

'Oi, Nightmare Nurse. You listening or what? Where are your manners?' Leroy laughed, then winced, grabbing onto his stomach.

'Easy, son,' said Barry. 'She's here to help.'

I bit my lip. 'Try not to strain yourself. I'd hate for you to rip your stitches. Only I'll have to stitch you up myself, given the shortage of surgeons.'

Leroy's face dropped.

'Extra-sharp needle.' I winked, laughing as he recoiled, that now familiar look of fear on his face. He thought he was a man, but it was clear, Leroy was just a boy. I'd seen him for what he was. Clearly, he didn't like it.

Barry cleared his throat. 'Nina, do you mind . . .'

Leroy kissed his teeth. 'Yeah, you heard the man. Run along now. Go disturb some other sick bastard.'

I cut Barry a look. 'Actually, I *do* mind. I mind very much. Visiting times are over. Not sure why you're here, Barry. This is a hospital, same rules apply for everyone, unless you've a good reason not to follow them?'

Barry snorted. 'I'll leave in a minute,' he said.

'Make sure you do,' I said.

The door closed behind me as I left the two men there, laughing at me behind my back. I felt my blood boil as I peered, once more, through the window. Their voices had quietened, but they were talking again – now in lower whispers. Barry was standing over Leroy, glancing at something on Leroy's phone. That sight of them together really made me burn. There was no way Leroy should be allowed to just lie there, getting away with what he did.

I moved into the corridor, calculating my movements. Ravi rushed past me then stopped dead in his tracks.

'Nina, hi.' His white coat was oversized, his body drowning in material. 'Wondered if I could have a minute?'

*I'd rather not.*

My stomach clenched. 'Of course. Let's go in here.'

I led him to the office, staring at the back of his skinny neck as he walked.

We entered the room and sat down. Ravi yawned, asking me to excuse his exhaustion.

'I was hoping to catch Barbara, but since you're around . . .' he said.

'What's all this about?'

He glanced around him, then leaned back in his chair, crossing his legs.

'No one here. It's private,' I said.

Ravi scratched his face. 'I've been doing a few checks, see. Comparing prescriptions with supply levels in each ward.'

'Right.' My heart began beating faster.

'It's something the new management are getting quite strict about. And . . . it's the numbers. They don't add up.'

I pinched my hands, attempting to act normal. 'What doesn't add up?'

'It's morphine. There seems to be an increase in sign-outs in the ledger. Not huge amounts – so no need to panic. But enough for me to notice. Sign-outs don't match prescribed levels. I thought I'd better mention it, so you can keep an eye out – make sure it's legit.'

I straightened up, desperately trying to appear professional.

'It might be nothing,' he said. 'But I'm obliged to look into it. Some of the names, the writing . . . looked a bit odd.'

'What do you mean?'

'Just similar across entries,' said Ravi, 'but the sign-out names were different.'

'I see.' I didn't like Ravi. He had a patronising tone. 'Well, I'm sorry. Can't help you. But I'll keep an eye out.'

'If you could, that would be great. I'll be monitoring things more closely from now on. We can review again next month.'

Ravi stood up, brushing his trousers down.

'That's all?' I asked.

'Actually. Could you talk to Barbara about it as well? I can never seem to catch her,' he said.

'She's busy. We all are.'

'Tell me about it. I'm flat-out. Yesterday, the queue outside the pharmacy was a mile long. That's on top of all the other administrative bits the management want. I'd better go.'

As he left, I felt my body deflate. I moved to the window to open it wide. I swallowed a mouthful of air, knowing this was the sign I needed – that I'd better get a hold of myself and not take any chances.

I finished my shift, worn and wearied by the busy night I'd just endured. I sent Mercedes a text and we agreed to meet for breakfast in the canteen. When she arrived, I didn't feel much like talking.

We moved to our preferred place at the back of the hall, carrying trays piled with scrambled eggs and toast. When we found a seat, Mercedes launched straight into an episode of the latest goings-on in maternity.

'So, there was this forty-five-year-old woman, well-to-do and all that. Proper posh accent. Fully dilated,' she said.

'Mmm . . .' I bit into my toast, picturing Ravi, irritated that he just couldn't leave it. And then there was Barry. *What a bloody cheek.*

'And I told her, you'd better start pushing because it's time.'

I nodded, forking scrambled eggs into my mouth. I couldn't speak to Barbara, I thought. I knew she would start digging.

'Well, she stops. Just like that . . .'

'Sorry, what?' Mercedes had my interest now.

'Says this wasn't part of the deal. "I don't want to do this," she says. "Fuck this. I've changed my mind."' Mercedes chuckled.

'Surely that's not how it works.' I lifted my mug, brought it to my lips. The steam brushed against my nose and provided comfort.

'By now, the baby's head is out, so of course, we all hold her down. She's screaming, and by God, can this woman scream. She's screaming like she's giving birth to a demon.'

I threw my head back and laughed. 'Then what?' I patted my mouth with a serviette, belly satisfied, spirits lifted.

'Just like that, she tries to get off the bed. Says she's going home and has had enough! But then, within seconds, the baby slips out.'

'Another normal day in maternity, then.' I was still smiling, but then I thought of Farah, what she'd said to me – too many post-birth fatalities that needed reporting to the public.

'I tell you, Nina, I don't know how much more of this I can take. What happened with the raid has really disturbed me . . . makes me more determined to get the hell out of here. I know I keep saying it but . . .'

I leaned back in my chair taking another sip of tea, adding more sugar when I realised I couldn't taste any.

'They're putting on an emergency community meeting to discuss what happened. Everyone is demanding we talk about it.'

I nodded. I'd got the alert from levinstonematters.com too, but after last time, I was not sure if I should attend. I was losing faith that anything would change.

'I need to ask you something,' I said, because now, that last conversation with Farah was playing on my mind again.

Mercedes looked up. 'What is it?'

'How did we get ourselves into a financial black hole, do you know? Where did all the money go? It's the reason we're under pressure and stretched so thin. We'll start making terrible mistakes and we'll be blamed unless it's filled.'

Mercedes looked down. 'I don't know. Things like that are kept quiet in management. Are you suspecting something a bit dodgy went on?'

'I don't know.'

Mercedes took a sip of coffee. 'Wouldn't surprise me. All the pressure departments are under. Richard says outsourcing is the answer, but it's causing more problems. Last thing we need is a new process and potential job cuts. Why are you thinking about this?'

'I'm thinking about a lot of things,' I said. 'We're having to run around to ensure the new process works for bloods. Plus, we're doing so many of them lately.'

'It's the same in maternity,' Mercedes said, thinking. 'But we've had more patients in, overall.'

'I don't know. Things just feel off,' I said.

'You should do some digging if you're worried. You're a head nurse and well respected.'

'Yeah. Maybe I should.' I should do something about it rather than just sitting still.

'Just bear in mind the RCN's negotiations are on everyone's mind. That is something good and positive to focus on. Fighting for better wages and patient safety. Helps get us the right attention.'

'True.'

'You are taking part, I assume?'

'Of course,' I said. It never crossed my mind *not* to be there with the others. But I was conflicted about haranguing the government for more money when there was a black hole, questions over how that money was spent. Plus, I needed money myself. I wasn't sure I'd be able to afford to go on strike.

'We all deserve better,' said Mercedes. 'It's not fair they don't pay us properly. I want to get out, maybe even settle down. When you mentioned Jacob the other day, it got me thinking about my life . . .'

But now, I was staring out of the window watching

families walk by. I was thinking of Farah, Ravi, Leroy, Dev. Balraj lying in that hospital bed.

Mercedes reached out her hand. 'Are you okay? You seem . . . lost. We haven't spoken since that incident on the bus.'

'I'm absolutely fine,' I said, but I felt a pang in my chest.

'Are you sure?' Mercedes squeezed my hand. 'Do you want to talk about anything?'

*Are you okay?*

Three little words that carried so much meaning. My eyes filled; my shoulders juddered. Mercedes rushed to the other side of the table and held me close to her.

# 12

Mercedes and I were fifteen when we first met. It was in Maple Tree Children's Home in West London, an unregulated home, disguised to look like every other smart Victorian semi to deter predators.

We'd arrived on the same hot summer's day in June 2010. Mercedes was there because her parents were alcoholics. I was returning to care after a failed foster-home placement. There's a certain bond that forms between girls who have no one left in the world to trust. That first day we met, our hearts opened to greet one another without fear or judgement.

We bumped into one another in the kitchen. I remembered how Mercedes first appeared: a beautiful Jamaican girl, cool and calm, cigarette in hand. Ripped jeans, a grubby Oasis T-shirt. She looked me up and down, figuring I'd probably do for now. A short, slightly podgy girl, with a shock of angry hair; I was incapable of doing her any harm.

Mercedes stubbed out her cigarette in a dirty coffee mug. 'How come you're in here?' she asked.

I wasn't sure what to say. In a place like this, I knew it was better to keep personal information private.

'*Come on.* You can say. I'm not like the rest of them. Besides, we're not so different. Jamaican?'

I figured I had nothing to lose. 'I'm half, Indian and Black. Not sure what kind.'

'Interesting.'

Mercedes looked like she'd had a rough time and, toughened, might offer me some protection.

'I was with a foster family, and it didn't work out. I don't know who my real parents are.' I'd relayed this story so many times, I sounded like I was describing adverse weather conditions.

'Found you difficult, did they?' She peered at me like it was a trick question.

'Not really.'

'So, you liked them, but they didn't like you?'

I also learned, early on, that Mercedes liked to ask a lot of questions.

'I wouldn't say that.' It didn't take long for me to blurt it all out. 'There was this woman . . . She made me do things . . .'

Mercedes' eyes glittered.

A care worker walked into the kitchen, carrying a heavy load of shopping. 'You've met one another, that's good. You'll need friends in here.' That was Russell Brompton, in charge. 'I tried to get you separate rooms, but you know how it is. Not enough single rooms for everyone.'

Mercedes tugged at my arm, bringing her face closer to mine. 'What things? What did she make you do?'

We scuttled into the hallway, running up the narrow stairwell. Catching sight of one another's bags in the same room on the second floor, we entered, crashing onto our beds. I scanned my new surroundings, my bed on the left as you walked in. Mercedes' bed was beside the window, next to a sink. There was a coffee stain on the blue carpet. I rubbed my arms. For some reason, I felt suddenly cold.

'Just chores around the house,' I said. *Get down on your hands and knees, you useless bitch. Scrub the floors clean to earn your keep.* 'The husband did a runner.'

'Fucking hell,' she said. Mercedes walked to the mirror to apply a thick coat of lipstick. 'Still, you're out of it now. We can look out for each other in here.'

I remember how my heart felt warm for the first time. What it meant to meet someone, a friend, during the darkest hours of my life.

'Why are *you* in here?' I asked.

'My parents are useless and drunk. Didn't look after me properly. My brother was lucky. He's five years older and got out. Lives with my uncle now.'

'And you couldn't go live with your uncle?'

'Not enough room. Plus, he looks at me funny.'

Mercedes fluffed her hair, tucking her T-shirt tightly into her jeans to accentuate her cleavage.

I nodded like I knew exactly what Mercedes meant, but I didn't, not really.

'Want to go out?' asked Mercedes. 'It won't do you any good staying cooped up in here.'

'Go where?' I looked Mercedes up and down. What struck me was that, although she was dressed like a teenager, her face, her voice appeared much older than her years. There was something wild and dangerous about her that dared me to go wherever she went but also warned me to be careful. 'I'm not sure. Curfew is seven thirty. It's our first night here. I don't want to get into trouble.' I sounded so self-righteous.

Mercedes burst out laughing. 'Well, that's up to you. Just lock the door, okay? I've got a key. If anyone asks, tell them I'm sleeping.'

Mercedes rolled her coat and stuffed it under her blanket. I felt an overwhelming urge to convince her to stay but knew it would be pointless.

'Want to go outside and smoke? At least tell me you smoke.'

'I don't smoke,' I said. 'I've never even tried it.'

'Jeez.'

Later that night, waiting for Mercedes to return home, I heard a car engine outside the window. My stomach rumbled from not eating enough, but as I listened more closely, I heard a man's voice, the clunk of a car door. Soon afterwards, someone crept up the stairs, but no one came to check who it was.

The door handle to our bedroom turned. I pressed my eyes tightly closed. Mercedes didn't say a word, at least, not on that first night. It was like both of us understood the rules of our friendship at the outset.

Mercedes slipped out of her clothes, brushing her teeth in the sink beside the window. I heard her gargle and spit, felt her shaky movements in the dark as she tucked herself under her duvet. She was breathing hard and fast, wriggling to make herself comfortable.

'Are you alright?' I whispered.

'I'm alright,' said Mercedes. 'I know what I'm doing.'

That night, after work, after she'd comforted me, Mercedes and I agreed to go out. We'd discussed how important it was to keep positive. Feeling calmer, I was looking for a distraction. I was thinking about the community meeting. How I ought to duck my head into church before meeting Mercedes in the pub.

I arrived in church fifteen minutes late and lingered at the back of the hall. The meeting was in full swing, and there I was, watching it play out like it was a debate in the House of Commons.

Manisha was there, shouting at Barry – much deserved – waving her hands about. 'You've previously said the situation was complex!' I was surprised she'd had time to attend, given the state Dev was in, still very much a patient at Newgate.

Barry squirmed. 'They moved on bikes. They were surprisingly fast, weaving through traffic. They were difficult to identify.'

*Bullshit, Barry. I gave you a video.*

'Well, that lady over there . . .' Manisha pointed to Grace, the schoolteacher who'd also spoken at the first meeting. '"Don't judge these youngsters," she said. But just look where we are now. How can we turn a blind eye when they've looted hard-working shop owners and stabbed an innocent man?'

I saw Grace's face burn. I could tell she hadn't expected to be singled out. Truth be told, I felt a bit sorry for her, being attacked publicly like that.

Grace stood up, her head firmly on her shoulders. 'I am not condoning their behaviour. I never said it was *acceptable*. All I said is that the *background* to how they got to this place is complex.'

'Restorative justice,' intoned Pastor Otis, 'that is surely

what is needed. It promotes healing and better dialogue. I say we invite these children into the house of God and we hear from them.'

That was when I left the church. The last thing I wanted was to come face to face with the town's tormentors. It was bad enough that no one had been arrested for stabbing Balraj.

It was seven o'clock by the time I arrived in the Fox and Hounds pub on the edge of Levinstone. Resting my elbows on the sticky bar counter, I ordered two gin and tonics, one for Mercedes, one for me. A friendly barman wearing hooped earrings rang my order. But I realised I couldn't afford to pay, so I immediately cancelled it.

'Sorry about that,' I said, 'I'd better wait for my friend. Can I just have a glass of tap water, instead?'

My cheeks burned.

He reassured me. 'I can stick it on a tab if you like. Too much of a pain to refund it.' He smiled as if to say *this happens a lot.*

I moved to the back of the pub, finding a seat on a comfortable sofa. The log fire beside me crackled and spat, orange and yellow flames dancing. I stared out of the window catching sight of a taxi veer into the pub car park. Sinking back into my seat, I sipped my G&T, the fizz tickling my throat as it slipped down.

Outside, mothers and fathers walked by, clutching their toddlers' hands. Others wheeled shopping trolleys, carrying boxes and oversized bags. A tall, slim man climbed up the pub's steps, a crop of spiky brown hair, faded blue jeans. He looked familiar, that walk, that slight hunch to his shoulders. But he was too quick as he came through the double doors. I didn't catch who it was.

Before long, Mercedes breezed in, negotiating the crowd at the bar. She made her way towards me and waved. I stood up to hug her. The curls of her hair smelled like coconut.

'I really need a drink,' she said. 'Been rushed off my feet. Did you get me one?'

'I added it to a tab . . .' I glanced down.

'Enough said.' She removed her coat, flung it to the side and took a seat in the armchair opposite me. Between us, a table. 'My treat. I'll sort it later.' She sat down, lifted her glass and took a generous gulp. But I couldn't take my eyes off the tall man leaning against the bar.

'*God*. This place is packed. Remember when it was just our haunt? Now there's every Tom, Dick, and Harry here from the hospital.'

'This is the nearest pub to Newgate,' I mumbled.

'No, it isn't. There's the Harvester. Why can't they all go there?'

I was transfixed, watching the man slide across the room, effortlessly cool. He stopped back at the bar and turned, scanning the tables. Our eyes locked and I smiled as it dawned, a warm sensation spreading, that it was Nikolaus, but with shorter hair. He'd obviously been to the barber's. My stomach flipped because now, as much as I loved Mercedes, I knew the evening was about to get more interesting. He turned and began chatting to the barman and ordered a pint.

I grabbed my drink, taking an extra-large sip, enjoying the lemony fizz on my top lip. Nikolaus raised and tilted his glass. I smiled again, feeling my thighs tingle. There was something about his casual manner, his disinterest in others, comfortable in his own space and skin, that I found immensely attractive.

'I'm really glad we did this,' I said. 'I needed it after the community meeting.'

Mercedes nodded. 'Too bloody right. I heard things kicked off – arguments about blaming the wrong people.'

She sighed as she snuggled back into her seat. 'Now, about what you asked me before, about Newgate. Have you found out anything? Because I've heard a few things.'

'What did you hear?' I leaned forward.

'I've heard where all the money's been going.'

'Where? Clearly not staff.'

'Mainly fines, I think, for missing NHS targets.'

'Anything else?' I asked.

'It's just a rumour, but apparently, Richard forced through outsourcing despite opposition from the rest of the management. Worse still, some suspect he might have some personal links with MediCentral.'

'No! That's outrageous,' I said. 'Where did you hear that? Are you sure?'

'Mary in procurement.'

Mercedes grabbed the pub menus propped up on the side. She glanced down, running her fingers over the food items. 'It's a fucking joke,' she said. 'He has no sensitivity to how much people are worried by it. It's a difficult climate as it is. People can't afford to lose their livelihoods. And then, him having links to a supplier! But it might just be a rumour. You can't always believe what Mary says.'

I drained my glass.

'All the violence in town is making things worse,' I said.

'Them coming into the hospital is straining an already strained service. We're missing targets because of them. He might have brought in MediCentral to speed things up, not just to save costs. Still. It wouldn't surprise me if he did call in favours from his own mates. Everyone's connected, aren't they?'

'Let's not read too much into it,' Mercedes said. 'Mary does like drama.'

'But if it's true, that's corrupt. He can't get away with it.'

Mercedes blinked. 'What about this stabbing? It's all over the news.'

'Just awful,' I said. 'How anyone could do that to Balraj, I don't know. Did I tell you I had a video? But, of course, Barry says he can't use it.'

'Let me see!'

I handed Mercedes my phone and she stared into the screen. 'It's grainy . . . but it's clearly SK, taking up beds in the hospital. More staff, like you said, is what we need. I tell you, I just need to save up a bit more and then I'm leaving.'

I nodded, but talk like that, of leaving Levinstone, was not something I wanted to hear. She was so well dressed, a figure-hugging black knitted outfit, cowboy boots, chunky gold earrings. Not like me, wearing a scrappy jumper and jeans. How different we were as women.

I glanced at Nikolaus from the corner of my eye, in need of a distraction. He was acting coy, not wanting to make it obvious that he couldn't stop staring at me.

I smiled to myself.

Mercedes swung her head round, then back, staring hard at me. 'Are you giving that bloke the eye?'

'No!'

She was laughing now. 'Nina, you've not paid *any* attention to this conversation. Don't think I haven't noticed.'

'I think I recognise him,' I said quickly.

'Who is he, then?'

'One of the porters from the hospital. A new one.'

'Can't say I've noticed him. Mind you, there are new porters each week. Newgate can't hold on to staff. Yet another problem.'

'His name is Nikolaus,' I said. My stomach fluttered just saying it.

'See you've done your homework, then.' Mercedes sniggered, circling her finger on the top of the table. 'Shall I order some food? Or maybe you'd like to go up there yourself and talk to *Nikolaus*. Skip the mains, darling. Go straight to the dessert.' She thought that was hilarious.

'Stop it,' I said, grabbing the menu.

The two of us settled on what to eat. Nikolaus had now disappeared; I was hoping he hadn't gone far. Mercedes traipsed to the bar and placed our order: a quinoa salad for me, scampi and chips for herself.

'I need to tell you something,' said Mercedes when she returned. She sat down and shuffled closer. 'Don't know if you've heard but a journalist has been sniffing around the hospital. Been asking all sorts. The management are apoplectic. There's an email due tomorrow, reminding people not to open their mouths.'

I sat up straight. 'Who?' I didn't want to tell Mercedes about Farah. It was too early. I had nothing on Newgate. After last time, I knew I'd need something with substance.

'A woman, I think. Works for *Levinstone Gazette*. I just hope she gets her story straight.'

I took a sip. 'Are you worried about that?'

'Me? No.' Mercedes pulled back. 'Why would I be worried?'

'Because I hear mortality rates are especially high in maternity. People won't understand about the overspend. Journalists will just focus on the failings and wind up the public.'

She blinked. 'Yeah, well. What do you expect? We're burned out, overworked, just like all nurses are in every department. Maternity is obviously high risk. There's a shortage of midwives. It's been well documented in the media.'

'Sorry, I didn't mean to accuse—'

'It's fine. I'm just a bit . . . defensive,' she said.

After a while, I told her how overwhelmed I felt. Had it not been for her, giving me a shoulder to cry on, I may have had a meltdown.

'Strikes. It's the only answer.' Mercedes checked her hair in the camera of her phone. 'Underfunding is not our problem. Whatever perm staff there are need paying – and properly. We've got to force the government's hand.'

'But striking is unlikely to sort out Newgate's black hole – or whatever caused it,' I said. 'Or people like Richard.'

'Yeah, but it's a matter of appreciation and principle for *us*.' Mercedes placed her phone on the table. 'Plus, it would mean that some of us don't have to find other ways to supplement our income. We need to be paid properly, Nina. The fact that we aren't, given the service we perform, is a national disgrace. I've seen patients left on trolleys for hours. Mothers in labour crying out in pain, squirming in soiled sheets, fully dilated.' Mercedes pursed her lips. 'Do you know, it was an assistant with me for the last ten deliveries? We don't even have proper midwives, that's how short-staffed we are.' Mercedes leaned forward. 'I heard one patient in A&E waited so long, he became dehydrated and drank the water from a vase of flowers!'

'No!'

'It makes me so angry because I never signed up for this, a life of neglect, everything second-rate.'

I didn't want to talk about work anymore. It was all too much. Besides, Nikolaus was back, and he'd just thrown me a smile.

The waiter brought our food, and by now, I was starving. I lifted my fork, tucking in. 'It's not always been this bad,' I said, munching.

Mercedes smiled. 'Do you remember Rob's retirement party when you got yourself stuck in that bin . . . When we hosted a Macmillan Coffee Morning, and were high on sugar for *days*?'

'What about the silent disco? That was weird.'

Mercedes checked her phone. '*Shit*,' she said.

'What is it?'

'Nothing.'

'*Tell* me.'

'It's just *her* – Sugar. Wants to know where I am and what I'm doing.'

I clenched my jaw. 'For crying out loud. Why now?'

Mercedes placed her phone down. I watched a woman next to us peel off her denim jacket.

'We have an arrangement. So that's how it is,' said Mercedes. 'I told you, it's not forever. I'm saving up enough so I can get out. Hopefully out of nursing as well.'

I dropped my fork onto my plate. The woman next to me sat up straight.

'Look, I've got to go speak to her,' she said. 'I can't keep her waiting.'

Before I could answer, Mercedes grabbed her bag to leave.

I stared down at her plate of food, still warm. I figured I'd better finish it for her. Through the window, I watched her pacing up and down the pavement. She had her phone pressed to her ear, a hand covering her mouth. I couldn't help but admire that at least Mercedes had somebody special in her life. She hung up and started to walk off.

I slumped back into the sofa, sipping my drink. The ice rattled around in my glass. When I looked up, Nikolaus was standing in front of me. I swallowed hard.

'Your friend is gone?' He smiled.

I noticed the adorable gap in his front teeth, aware that I was now alone and ready for the evening. 'Yeah, she's gone.'

His smile widened as he sat down opposite, staring at me with his brilliant green eyes. 'It is good to see you again,' he said. 'You look beautiful tonight.'

My heart skipped a beat. I glanced out of the window, watching the back of Mercedes. *God*, I hoped she would not be returning.

'You were working today?' he asked.

'Yes. But I'm off tonight.'

He smiled. 'Me, also. I return in the afternoon, tomorrow.'

He leaned forward, pressing his palms flat on the table. I

scanned his hands. Definitely no wedding ring. Lovely clean fingernails.

His eyes flickered mischievously.

'How long have you been working at the hospital?' I asked, trying not to make it so desperately obvious how hot I suddenly was. Just seeing Nikolaus sitting there was enough to make me hungry to learn every little detail about him. I stared at his hands once again, his fingers, thick and long. His wrists, with tufts of soft brown hair sprouting from under the cuffs of his shirt.

'I start as a porter, but from today, they move me to the mortuary.'

I didn't think too much about it. Of course, now I see how significant that was, how integral to the outcome of what happened later.

Outside the window, Mercedes was now fumbling around in her handbag.

'I get more drinks,' he said, and he stood up. 'Whiskey?'

'Sure, why not.'

I watched his back turn, trying to figure out what it was about him that made him feel so different. He ordered two tumblers of neat whiskey at the bar, and I used the quiet moment to send Mercedes a text.

*If you need to leave, don't worry. Nikolaus is chatting me up at the table!*

Mercedes instantly replied:

*Still on the phone. Sugar having a showdown with her husband. He found my messages!*

Nikolaus returned, handing me a glass. The drinks were stronger than I'd expected, and I winced as the whiskey went down. 'Are you sure those are doubles?'

'Maybe triple.' He laughed.

'Surely illegal!'

'I know Georg the barman.'

It did not take long for my bones to thaw, for the air between us to sweeten and warm.

'So, where are you from, originally?' I asked. I was imagining taking him back to my flat, ripping off his clothes, scratching his back.

He gulped a large mouthful. 'It is complicated. But I tell you everything. Basically, I am from Germany. I move to UK with my friend, Stefan, also German. We try to find some work. Levinstone is cheap, so it is perfect for us.'

'It's great you have a friend. Moving to London can be lonely.'

He smiled. 'We are very close. Like brothers.'

'That's wonderful. I have Mercedes. My best friend. We moved here together, too. Known each other since childhood.' I sighed. 'But Levinstone is going downhill.'

'Downhill?'

'Getting rough, too much crime. An English expression.' Someone had turned on the jukebox. It meant I had to shout.

Nikolaus nodded, taking another sip. 'I heard about what happened to the man,' he said. 'It's terrible. Where I live, in Germany, it is not so different.'

I bit my lip.

'I was born in UK but moved around,' I said. 'I arrived here when I was studying to be a nurse. Do you know the

Training College of Nursing and Midwifery? It's in the nicer part of town.'

Nikolaus nodded.

'That is where I was.'

He raised his eyebrows. It felt good to know I'd impressed him.

'Are you with someone?' he asked after a while. No forewarning. Straight to the point. I figured it was something to do with German directness.

'I haven't connected with anyone in the way I'd like to.' I tried hard not to sound so available.

He grinned. 'Me too.'

From that moment on, more alcohol flowed. Nikolaus told me stories of his time in Heidelberg. 'You know, I was a little wild. A man always in trouble . . .'

The sounds of the other punters rose and fell, and soon, we grew aware only of each other among the crowds. The electricity between us crackled like the flames of the log fire. Heidelberg sounded strangely musical. After a quick image search on Google, I found it was beautiful as well. This man was a lovable rebel, with exactly the right kind of restless mischief I adored. Just what I needed to lift me from the darkness of Leroy. Barry. Newgate Hospital.

Before long, I found myself clambering into a cab, giggling so hard, my stomach hurt.

The cab pulled away from the kerb. I lowered the window, enjoying the cold air against my cheeks, closing my eyes as I inhaled deeply.

'A small-time German life is not for me. I came to London for an adventure, Nurse Nina!' He stroked my cheek.

I rested my head on his shoulder and breathed in the scent of him: woody with caramel, mixed in with cigarettes and petrol.

I was desperate to know what might happen between us. I really liked this man. I was attracted to him in a way I could not explain. Just being in his presence was beautiful and strangely . . . enough.

As the cab threaded through traffic, the street lights dripped and streaked in front of my eyes. Buildings turned into flats, flats into houses, houses into shops. In my mind's eye, hospital beds flashed. I saw Dev, Leroy and, surprisingly, Barry's concerned face.

The cab slowed as we pulled up outside my flat. Like a gentleman, Nikolaus paid the driver and eased me out of the back. As we stood on the pavement, he looked up and laughed.

'A samosa shop!' he sang.

We stumbled into my flat, tripping up the stairs.

Only for a second did it occur to me that this was dangerous. I didn't know this man – not really. Could I trust him not to hurt me? In a certain shade of light, others might think him strange.

He peeled off his jacket and shirt, leaving on a white vest. I felt a rush of adrenalin, a yearning to feel his flesh. An overwhelming urge to bite into his skin.

'Your flat is very small but nice,' he said, glancing around him. He neatly folded his shirt, placing it on the bed. I didn't need to tell him how important it was that he tidy up after himself. 'A studio,' he said, 'is it enough room for you?' Before I could stop him, he was pulling off his vest.

I held my breath as he wandered over to the shelves in his jeans, belt unbuckled, naked from the waist up. Hair sprouted in the outline of a tree. Bushy across the chest, a thin trunk leading down to his stomach and circling his belly button.

He peered at the framed photos on the shelf.

'That's one of me, when I graduated from college.' I moved closer, my cheek brushing against his shoulder. I felt his skin, warm and soft.

'All nurses just like you.' He laughed. 'And your family . . . where are they?'

The alcohol in my system seemed to dull just then. I stepped back, my body heavy, as I moved to the bed and sat down on the edge.

'Do you want more to drink?' I whispered. I knew I had a bottle somewhere.

He turned, silently, then sat down next to me.

I moved closer to him, and he draped an arm around me, kissing my forehead. 'I do not have a family,' he said. 'I was left alone. To this day, I do not know who, or where they are.'

I looked up at him without blinking, my heart in my mouth.

'I was cared for by a teacher in my village,' he said.

He was someone just like me, wandering through life, lost and empty.

'Are you serious?' I whispered.

He nodded, drawing me closer.

'I have not told anyone except my friend Stefan.'

'It's the same for me,' I breathed. 'It's too painful to talk about, isn't it?'

He lifted my chin and brought his lips closer to mine. I closed my eyes and felt myself surrender.

After that kiss, we did nothing but hold each other in the warmth of the darkness, offering each other comfort and reassurance.

Soon we drifted off to sleep, traversing and exploring worlds together, laughing in our dreams. We wailed like feral wolves. The alcohol helped me to forget, melting my bones, easing my muscles. Inside myself, I felt like I was lost, and yet, now, I'd found someone special. Nikolaus was abandoned like me. That alone felt like a miracle. It had taken a lifetime for me to find someone who had the capacity to understand life as I'd known it. Someone who could love me just as I was, with so many parts of myself missing.

The next morning, a beautiful silver light filled the living room. My eyes slowly adjusted as I realised it must be Diwali. I turned and saw that Nikolaus had left me a note. I hauled myself up onto my elbows.

*Nina, I cannot tell you how happy I am that I have found you. Thank you for a wonderful night. I hope you will call me or see me in the hospital. I have a very early morning shift. My colleague is sick, and they ask me to work. I did not want to disturb you. I am very sorry not to say goodbye. But I want to see you again. If nothing else, I just want us to be friends. xxx*

Something in me felt like I'd been given a second chance.

# 13

That night, I cared for my patients with renewed focus and energy, catching up on my notes, assisting patients onto the toilet. But it was naïve to think it would last.

I moved to the next patient on my list, Dev, and hoped he might be feeling better. I saw Manisha rush past, slamming her hand against the exit button.

In the bay, enveloped in a warm, comforting haze, Dev lay on his side, his back towards me. The air was peaceful and light. A vase full of water stood on the table containing a lone tangerine-coloured gerbera daisy tilted to one side. Manisha's slippers lay in the corner, her cream cardigan slung on the back of a chair.

'Mum's not here,' Dev whispered, his voice breathy. 'It's Diwali . . .'

'I know,' I said. 'I saw her leave. She'll be back soon. I imagine she's delivering sweets.'

His eyes remained closed. I checked his notes and saw that he had been overseen by Sandra and a nurse from Platinum Care earlier. They'd carried out three more FBCs since my last shift, which was strange. Yesterday, one at 9 a.m., 9 p.m., and then another at 9 a.m. this morning. The CT scan had also returned – all normal.

'Nurse . . . I've done so many tests. Is it possible that the bloods are . . . wrong?'

I thought for a moment. 'It's highly unlikely and if the

FBCs aren't showing anything, there would be no reason to worry.'

'But it *is* . . . possible?'

Of course it was possible. Anything was possible. I carried out the usual obs then tried to distract myself by tidying up around him. I folded Manisha's cardigan and replaced it on the spare chair. Marg and Colin were asleep, which was just as well.

'I've been making some plans . . . just in my head . . . for when I get out,' whispered Dev.

'Sounds great. Good to have a plan.'

'I'm going to write . . . an album.'

I glanced at him and smiled. He needed to get out, to go and live his life.

'And there's this girl . . . I've been seeing her for two years. She's black. Mum won't allow it . . . but I'm ready to take it to the next level.'

'*You* like her. That's all that matters.'

I sat down, my head feeling lighter. Young love was beautiful.

'Aaliyah . . . proper gorgeous, she is. I'm going to marry her . . . one day.'

I leaned forward, placing my hand on his. 'Sounds like a fairy tale. Don't worry about what your mum thinks.'

'"You can marry anyone but a black girl," that's what she said. But life's too short . . . to listen to talk like that . . .'

Dev coughed and placed a hand on his stomach.

I swallowed hard, thinking of the two disparate sides of me. I imagined Dev and Aaliyah together, as parents, raising a child. They'd probably make a success of things. Be accepted for the lovely people they are. But look at me: split down the middle.

I wondered what Nikolaus was doing.

'I'm going to take life seriously from now on,' said Dev. 'No more messing about . . .'

I knew exactly what he meant – that time is short, with no guarantee of what might happen next. It was impossible to be a nurse, confronted with the fragility of life, and not think about how, each day, we are all approaching the end. Wasting so much time, worrying over little things.

'You're a good nurse.' He sighed. 'You're not like the others. I haven't been good . . . I'm not the son my mum thinks I am . . .'

I could tell he was drifting, his words growing faint and jumbled.

I stood a little unsteadily and stared down at the outline of him. 'No one is perfect, Dev. I wouldn't beat yourself up about it.' I was about to leave through the gap in the blue curtains, but Dev said something more.

'Nurse . . .' His voice was weak, breathless. Something in it was different.

'How can I help?'

'Last night . . . I heard flutes playing.'

'Flutes, did you say?'

'Just subtle notes . . . like the ones you sometimes hear in Hindu temples. It felt so . . . peaceful.'

I stepped forward, wiping a stray hair from his brow, beaded with sweat. I brought my face closer to his, to take a good look at him.

'What does it mean?' I asked.

'I don't know, it just felt . . . important. Because, you know, it's Diwali.'

I pulled away. 'When the doctor passes, I'll be sure to mention it.'

The buzzer went off in Leroy's room. Annoying as it was, I had no choice but to see what he wanted.

It was quiet inside Leroy's room. I waited beside the door, watching him stir, growing aware of my presence.

His eyes flickered and opened.

'What do you want?' I asked, standing beside him in the dark.

'Finally,' he groaned. 'I need water . . .'

I glared at him, this pathetic creature. I moved to the sink, pouring water from the tap. I returned to his bed, handing him the cup.

'Leave it on the side, will ya?'

I bit the inside of my cheek, placing the cup on the table. 'Anything else?'

He stirred, slowly rearranging himself so that he now lay flat on his back, a hand resting on his thigh, his cannula in the skin of the dorsum of his hand. He stared up at me, then fixed his eyes on a spot on the ceiling.

'What is it with you?' he said.

I scoffed, not in the mood to engage in a deep and meaningful conversation with a criminal. Certainly not wanting to ruin the first good day and night I'd had in ages. 'I know who you are, I know what you did. I'm sure Barry knows too – that's the reason why you've got away with it.'

He thought for a few seconds. 'You think I'm part of a gang, like them other guys terrorising this town.'

'And you're not?'

Leroy lowered his eyes and glanced at me.

'Barry should know better,' I said.

He scoffed. 'You're too judgemental, you need to chill. You're no different to me. You don't even *know* me, so how you passing judgement?'

There was no point standing there, talking to him. I felt a tug at my core that I ought to check on Dev, was even convinced that I'd heard him coughing in the distance. But Leroy kept going on and on.

'You're half Jamaican, right?'

'I don't know.'

'What do you mean, *don't know*? I can tell. How come you can't?'

My chest felt tight. 'If there's nothing else . . .' I walked away, determined not to let him get the better of me. Men like Leroy never learned. They were entitled, stubborn, pig ignorant. Desperate to cut good people down.

'You're half something else, though. Indian, is it? That side pulling a bit harder? Must be confusing, having two sides. Split personality, even.'

I walked out. I didn't want to listen to him anymore.

I went to see if Dev was awake. I needed to carry out obs, but was aware I was running a few minutes late. Leroy was getting to me.

'Dev?'

I stood over him, peering into his eyes. The lids were wide open, the black dots of his pupils dilated, the whites veiny with blood.

'Can you hear me?' I shook him a little.

His face was vacant, so I leaned closer, spotting a trickle of vomit from his mouth, staining the pillow. I shook him more forcefully, desperate for any response or signs of life. His body was scraggly and floppy like a rag doll.

Airway, vomit. Breathing, none. Circulation, disability, exposure . . . Panic rose. I had only just left him. I immediately went to work, scooping out the waste from his airway. Applying a mask to him. Delivering breaths from an Ambu bag, pumping hard.

'Dev, talk to me. C'mon. Dev!'

But there was nothing.

Anchored to the floor, bile fizzing in my stomach, the rush of overwhelm made it difficult to act fast enough. Thoughts jumbled.

'Dev . . . please!'

I heard Marg and Colin stir. 'What's happening?' mumbled Marg. 'Why all the noise?'

Dev did not move. His body was silky smooth, creamy, like a wax figure. His mouth was open, as if the last word he'd meant to say was still lodged in his throat. For the first time, I noticed his long lashes, his delicate fingers. His hand clenching a ball of bedding, a gesture fixed and frozen.

I saw in Dev's face the blank pages of music we'd only just discussed he'd create.

I sounded the alarm – calling for help.

While the others came running, I rushed to the front desk to call for the doctor. I recalled seeing Dr Milburn rushing down the corridor, stomach wobbling, tie rippling. I remembered the soft slapping sound his soles made against the vinyl floor.

The others arrived seconds later. Frantically, they began chest compressions. I stood back, unable to move. I watched Preeti apply defib pads to Dev's chest in search of a heart rhythm, hopeful that perhaps the shocks might reverse the cardiac arrest.

But the room soon fell silent.

All the lessons I'd received on how to deal with a patient in a moment like this dissolved. Dev was gone. He was a wisp, a gentle breeze, passing through the clotted air, throughout the ward, the labyrinth of the hospital.

As the others walked into the corridor, heads down, I moved to the window, struggling to open it. A psychic force rushed from behind me, escaping through the glass. A second of silence passed before a breeze rushed forward.

What happened next is a blur. No matter how many times I go over it in my mind, I'm unable to remember precisely what happened.

'I'm sure you did all you could,' Dr Milburn said, a mumble of voices now surrounding him. He stood next to Barbara, discussing, in hushed voices, how to keep this latest episode low-key.

'We had better take over from here,' Barbara said. 'The notes, Nina. Where are they?'

I sat down on a chair in the corridor, rocking back and forth, the crampy pain in my stomach unlike anything I'd ever experienced before.

They kneeled beside me as I updated them on Dev's condition. He was fine, I pleaded, *absolutely fine*!

'Has anyone called the mother?' asked Barbara. 'We need to call her now.'

But at that precise moment, Manisha arrived back on the ward. A strong scent of sandalwood trailed behind her. She let out a guttural cry, a howl from the deepest part of her, clambering onto the bed, clawing at the sheets, screaming – grabbing onto Dev. The red bindi on her forehead smeared as she begged for one more chance to feel him against her skin. Security guards rushed in to restrain her. They grabbed her shoulders, her waist, because she fought, my God, she fought hard, no power in this world strong enough to keep mother and son apart.

They won. Manisha stumbled to the floor, dry retching next to her son's trainers and cross-body satchel. 'Murderers! You are all murderers!'

Those were the last words I heard as I left the ward.

# 14

I was given a day off to recover, armed with a brown envelope stuffed with leaflets advertising helpline numbers. But later that afternoon, having given up on the prospect of getting any decent sleep, bored from aimlessly surfing TV channels to stop myself reliving that scene, I picked up a copy of the *Levinstone Gazette* to skim-read an article:

> *Diwali delight for British Asians as Rishi Sunak becomes UK PM.*

Farah had quoted Rishi's first speech as prime minister:

> *This government will have integrity, professionalism, and accountability at every level . . . Trust is earned. And I will earn yours . . . A stronger NHS. Better schools. Safer streets . . .*

I swallowed, my throat sore. It was the stress of Dev's death, taking hold of me like tonsillitis. All I kept thinking was, how could he have died?

A slow panic began to sweep over me. What if they found out I'd taken Dev's morphine tablets, all twelve of them, prescribed by Dr Milburn? Worse still, that box of thirty I'd swiped from the medical supplies cupboard? It was not as if I was addicted. I'd only ingested once. But now I could see that the risk I'd taken was disproportionately huge versus the benefit it offered.

I knew Maria had been asked to step in, to interview everyone involved during the mandatory seventy-two-hour internal investigation. She was, in my view, the worst possible person to manage this.

My stomach growled. I realised I hadn't eaten all day. To make matters worse, my fridge and cupboards were almost empty. I left my flat to stock up, and to distract myself.

The pavements were wet, the air muggy from rain. In the distance, a queue was forming outside the Shree Ram Hindu Temple and Community Centre. Inside they promised a week's worth of food. But only if you could provide an electronic voucher confirming a legitimate referral that you were in desperate need. With fourteen million people in the UK poverty-stricken, there was no shame in being here, they said. I had applied for one last week but was denied. But that didn't deter me.

I entered, overpowered by the scent of masala incense and colourful flowers, and spoke to a woman at the front desk called Savita.

'Can you prove you're in need?' she said.

I fumbled around in my pockets. 'Shit, I can't find it, but trust me, I'm a nurse and really *do* need this . . .'

She stared at me pensively, then broke into a smile. 'Oh, go on, then. It's Diwali. It's bad karma if you're lying.'

*Bad karma,* I thought. I'd already had my share.

She handed me a brown cardboard box. 'Next time, bring proof.'

I nodded, walking inside the main hall, green crates,

shelves and boxes stocked with essentials. I sifted through mini boxes of cornflakes, rice crispies, selecting a couple of cans of soup, kidney beans, packets of pasta, white rice fragranced with jasmine. I was grateful for the cartons of exotic juice and long-life UHT milk – maximum allowed, three of each. But I requested more cleaning products for my box. Always useful. A volunteer named Sharon did not hesitate to offer me a selection of cheap copycat brands. I grabbed a packet of sanitary towels on the way out, easily the most expensive item of the lot. I returned home just as the sky darkened, collapsing on the sofa with tiredness.

Mercedes sent me a text shortly afterwards, offering her usual advice:

*Fuck them. Like they haven't enough of their own failings across the board. They've no shame when it comes to blaming nurses. We don't get paid enough!*

I scanned the leaflets fanned out on the table, including the information offered on how to access support from within the hospital. I was about to call the Royal College of Nursing to check the finer details of my indemnity insurance, but I saw that Nikolaus had sent me a text. I must have missed it while messaging Mercedes.

*Nina! I hope I see you at work. When is your next shift? To be very honest, I cannot stop thinking about our night together. X*

I typed a reply:

*In tomorrow. Can't wait to see you then. X*

I knew that Nikolaus would be the best distraction of all.

The following evening, as I began my journey to work, the air was dark and oppressive. Walking along the dirty pavements, I caught sight of the red bus in the distance. I lifted the collar of my coat, fumbling around in my bag for my Oyster card. When the headlights drew nearer, I felt a hand firmly press down onto my shoulder.

'Manisha—'

She'd appeared out of nowhere, a light extinguished from her eyes, her cheeks hollow and sunken. She wore a shabby grey coat like a bathrobe. Her face was worn, like she hadn't slept in days.

She grabbed me more forcefully.

'Hey! What are you doing?'

'*You!*' she spat. Her voice hissed venomously like a snake. No matter how much I wanted to run, there was an invisible force keeping me there.

'You were supposed to be looking after him!'

'I'm so sorry – really I am.'

'How can you live with yourself?'

My legs trembled. 'What do you mean?' I said. 'I did everything I could – it wasn't my fault. We'd carried out every possible test and found nothing!'

'You – *you* are responsible, do you know that? *You* neglected my son. What – or *who* – was so important that you could not keep an eye on him?'

I felt my head rush. I told myself that what happened to Dev had nothing to do with me. I tried my best – *really*, I did. I did not, in a million years, ever foresee he would die. Did Manisha not remember how I ran around him all night?

*Leroy . . .*

'I told you all *so many times* . . . something is *wrong*, something is *wrong*.' Manisha's voice broke, her bottom lip quivered. 'But none of you listened. None of you took it seriously.'

'You have to believe me when I say I did everything I could . . .' My eyes lowered.

Manisha scoffed. 'Well, *could* isn't good enough. Presumably you don't have children of your own – you're too young. You'll never understand what a loss like this feels like.'

I moved to the edge of the pavement as the bus pulled up. The door opened and several passengers boarded. Manisha's gaze fixed onto mine, her retinas burning a hole in my eyes.

'They told me you were tending to another patient when you should have been looking after Dev. Is that true? Did you neglect him?'

'Of course not! Don't listen to gossip.' I closed my stinging eyes, unable to hear any more.

'He had everything going for him. I wanted him to settle down, to see him have children . . . to be the success I know he was destined to be. But you took that away. And all because you were *distracted*!'

'Listen to me—' I was desperate, glancing back and forth between Manisha and the bus. The doors were open; at any second, they would close. 'I did everything I could – *everything* to get him seen to. He did not even call me! I was with another patient who also needed me, but that was for like, a few minutes. No nurse can be with a patient twenty-four hours.'

But maybe Dev did call out. Maybe I didn't hear him.

I hesitated.

There was no way I could have heard him because I was preoccupied. That *idiot* Leroy. I'd wasted valuable time in what was, clearly, a critical moment. Had Leroy not called for me that night, expecting me to drop everything to see to him, I would have been there for Dev.

'I wasn't there . . .' Manisha said.

'It wasn't your fault either,' I whispered. 'Please don't blame yourself. It wasn't anyone's fault but . . .'

*Leroy.* When resources are stretched, it's outrageous he'd received treatment at all.

'Excuse me!' the driver called. His voice cut into the dark. 'Are you getting on this bus, or not?'

I reached out my hand and placed it onto Manisha's shoulder. She slapped it away, snarling like an angry wolf. 'Don't think you will get away with this. Don't think that you can continue your life as normal as if nothing's happened.'

'Manisha, please—'

'You will *pay*. Do you hear me? You will pay for your mistakes.'

'Oi, nurse! Not being funny, but you're holding everyone up!'

Her eyes bulged. 'Nothing you can do will ever bring him back. He was the only thing I had left worth living for, with the potential to do so much good in the world.'

'What good will come from blaming me?' I cried. 'There is a formal investigation. You will see the outcome for yourself.'

I turned, pleading for the bus to wait, waving my hands to signal that Manisha was a little crazy.

'Now!' said the driver. 'You're holding everyone up!'

I moved away from her.

'You said you would help me,' Manisha's voice trailed. 'You said he was safe!'

The doors closed behind me as I stepped onto the bus.

'But you failed him!'

I was relieved as the engine purred and rolled under my feet. My eyes to the floor, I avoided the angry stares of the other passengers.

I staggered down the aisle, past seats, brushing arms and shoulders. I grabbed onto the metal handrail as the bus drove along the road.

Through the steaming window, I saw Manisha standing at the bus stop, staring out into the road. As I took a seat at the back of the bus, that image of her still firmly lodged in my mind, I wondered if my own mother or father ever searched for me that way. Of course, I forgave her for behaving like that, a natural reaction to pain. She didn't mean any harm. I'd seen it so many times: shock and denial, grief turning to guilt, the angry blaming of others in the early stages of bereavement.

I pressed a hand against the window, silently pleading to Manisha to forgive me. My eyes streamed as the bus meandered through traffic.

In the hospital, I drifted into the canteen, swearing under my breath because I desperately wanted coffee and the machine was out of order. I moved to the side counter, fumbling around for a teabag nestled among discarded sugar wrappers, mini milk pots. I felt a tap on my shoulder. I jumped for a second, thinking it was Manisha, following me all the way here to scream at me again. But it was Nikolaus, his face beaming bright like a fresh, spring day, revealing an inner joy, a spiritual radiance which I hadn't noticed about him before.

'I am so happy to see you,' he said.

My heart skipped. Seeing him standing there, in his black T-shirt and jeans, I forgot, if only for a moment, the awful start I'd had to the evening. The black against his pale skin made the green in his eyes more vivid. I wanted to grab him, to sink my face into his chest, to nestle in the comfort of his chin. But I couldn't move.

'Hi,' I said sheepishly.

*Pathetic.*

'I'm sorry I left so quickly. You saw my note, yes?' he asked.

I nodded.

He leaned forward, brushing the hair out of my eyes. The touch of his fingertips took me back to that night we had.

'How are you?' It was all I could think to say.

'I'm fine.' He moved his hand and placed it on my lower back. 'I would like to see you again, Nina,' he said. He leaned closer. 'I cannot stop thinking about you.'

I caught the scent of his breath, faded tobacco and peppermint. But as I closed my eyes, Manisha's face appeared, boring into my brain.

I stepped back, my heart stuttered in my chest. 'I'm just a bit busy right now . . .'

His face fell.

'Look, about the other night—' I said.

'You do not want to see me?' He searched my face, searched for an explanation.

'It's not that. I'm just not used to this expectation, that's all.'

'Expectation?'

'I need some time . . . space to think.'

He swallowed, taking a step back. He simply nodded.

The air grew tense. I felt like a cold-hearted bitch. But a man had just died, and it was clear, yet again, I was fucking things up badly. It's what I usually did each time it seemed like I was moving forward.

'I'd better go,' I said quickly, walking away. Something in my heart hurt, but I did not allow myself to turn.

# 15

I stood over Leroy in the dark, watching him sleep. He was like a child dozing peacefully after drinking a heavy bottle of milk. This man, this *criminal*, had no regard for the grief he'd caused. I wondered what would happen if I stabbed him with a pair of sharp scissors.

Why was it that this monster lived, when an innocent – talented – young man had died, with the melody still left inside him?

*Manisha . . .*

How could it be that resources were poured on those least worthy when they were already so limited? I believed in the principle of free healthcare, but here, nothing made sense. No one told Leroy to join a gang. To be a thug, deal in drugs, cause mayhem. I toyed with the idea that no one would know if I killed him by mixing a concoction of medicines, if plunging a pair of scissors into his heart was considered too violent. No one would miss him because his contribution was small. If there was one thing I'd learned, it was that people died every second of every day. As harsh as it sounded, what difference would *his* death make?

Had Leroy not distracted me that night, with his constant whining and attention-seeking, Dev might still be alive. Why was it that the doctors prioritised him over a good man?

Because of Leroy, I could end up getting struck off as a nurse. Manisha would complain and my life would be over.

Something needed to happen to ensure Leroy received an appropriate punishment.

I stared at Leroy, this lowly creature, this sorry excuse for a man.

He stirred, then opened his eyes.

'Who's there?' He scanned the dark for an outline. 'What do you want?' he said, his voice quivering.

I moved closer, the warm metal of the scissors pressed into my palm.

'Nurse, is that you?'

I stood silently, listening to his voice rise and falter. It was time to give this waste of space a taste of his own medicine.

'What is it, for fuck's sake. Don't just stand there! Don't think I don't know it's you. You're a psycho, do you know that? Creeping up on me. What the hell do you want?'

I slid to the foot of the bed, lifting his notes. I clicked on a mini torch as I leafed through them. His wound was gaining strength, drying, visible signs of new tissue. But Leroy still needed heavy doses of painkiller.

'Poor little you.' I moved towards him, imagining all the ways in which I might hurt him: pulling out his cannula, stabbing him in the neck. Grabbing the pillow from under his head and pressing it hard onto his face. Every evil thought felt good, as if wires crossed and welded in my brain, fusing good and evil.

'Is everything okay?'

Sandra was standing there, staring at me in the dark. She flicked on the light. 'I heard voices, so I came to check everything was alright.'

I squinted as my eyes adjusted, waiting for the red dots

to disappear. When I opened them, I realised Sandra was staring directly at me.

I was perspiring.

'It's not okay! Let me tell you, yeah! This woman is a psycho. Get her away from me!' Leroy writhed in his bed, the plastic covering his mattress crinkling as his legs moved. 'I want to complain. She just stands there in the fucking dark for no apparent reason. It's intimidating.' He held on to his side and groaned.

'I was about to carry out obs,' I said dismissively.

Sandra lowered her eyes and nodded. 'Of course.'

I stepped away from him, wiping my clammy hands on my scrubs.

'I can take over if you like,' offered Sandra, more of an instruction than a recommendation. As she approached, I remember resenting being told what to do by *her*. Who did this woman think she was? Only the other day, it was *me* helping *her* out. Yet now, here she was, assuming authority over me that she hadn't earned.

'Does he need anything?' she asked.

'A dose of pain relief in an hour.'

She nodded.

'Good riddance!' shouted Leroy as I left the two of them alone. I closed the door gently behind me and bit hard on my tongue.

I knew I'd gone too far. I needed to get a grip.

I moved to the bathroom and stared hard in the mirror at the woman I'd become. As I watched the vein under my left eyebrow throb, I asked myself, *What am I doing?* I slipped into a cubicle in the far-right corner and securely locked the door.

This was ridiculous. I couldn't be seen like this. I needed to calm the fuck down. I was becoming a liability on the ward; I already knew that.

Certainly, there was a wound far deeper in me than I had imagined, affecting my demeanour. Not a wound caused by others, nor the accidental slash of my own skin, where I saw the fleshy gore inside, the raw nerves and ropy tendons. It was the bleeding wound inside myself, a tear in the deepest part of my soul. Most would say, upon hearing my story, that this wound was in my heart because that's ordinarily where we expect the deepest wound to be. But it was not there, it was in my stomach. The shock of losing Dev, that confrontation with Manisha, festering.

I'd swallowed the pain like a bitter pill, and now it had travelled down my oesophagus into the slimy cavern of my stomach. Gastric juices liquefied the lumpy mess of it all, digesting, then pushing it out, six metres, through my small intestine. There, it must have finally absorbed because my wound, my pain, had become impossible to ignore. Some good things were happening to me, of course. Nikolaus being one. His appearance in my life, opportune, karmic even. But Dev's death – and just now, my behaviour with Leroy – had the power to destroy it.

I felt a sudden urge to pee. Staring at the grey floor, I was about to go when the doors in the main area of the washroom opened. Two women entered; I recognised their voices. One belonged to Sandra. The second, breathy and hurried, was Barbara's.

'It's just a bit strange, that's all. I'm almost sorry to mention it.' That was Sandra.

'Not at all,' Barbara said. 'If you're worried about her, you must say. She's obviously upset, perhaps even a bit disturbed after what happened to Dev.'

'She was always the strong one, y'know?' said Sandra, her voice now conceited. 'I guess it's all been too much. Just goes to show what can happen . . .'

'But intimidating Leroy like that,' said Barbara. 'I must say, it's so unlike her, so disappointing.' The taps turned on; water splashed around the basins. 'I must address it before it gets any worse.'

There they were, discussing me as if I was a threat on the ward, a casualty of stress. Unfit to work. They'd implied I was compromising vital care. That was what cut me the most. What a cheek for Sandra to suggest I'd done anything wrong. All she'd seen me do was stand there in the dark. It enraged me to hear them say such nasty, spiteful things. Whatever happened to support, friendship, and camaraderie when fellow nurses needed it?

The hand dryers turned on; I struggled to hold my bladder.

'I can keep an eye on her if you like,' said Sandra.

'Oh, if you could, that would be great. You can be my eyes and ears while I'm submerged in paperwork. There appears to be no end to the admin, what with MediCentral coming in.'

'Of course!' said Sandra. I could almost see her gloating. 'Anything I can do. Just say the word.'

In the corridor, I returned to the front desk and sat down, briefly scanning the all-staff email reminding us that we were not permitted to talk to journalists. I rolled my eyes and slipped my hand into my pocket. My fingers pinched a small round tablet. Fuck it, what did I care what Sandra and Barbara thought about me? I prised the tablet out, placed it on my tongue and swallowed hard. I wanted to enjoy how my body relaxed.

I was about to go on a twenty-minute break, so I sent Nikolaus a text, asking him to meet me in the canteen because now I regretted how cold I'd been. Here was a man who'd said he cared for me, who liked me just as I was. And there *I* was, a total idiot.

In the canteen, the air smelled of boiled cabbage. I walked in, floating, almost, unable to feel my feet. Nikolaus shuffled in, sheepish, hands wedged in his jeans. He must've thought I was one of those women messing about with him.

'I just wanted to say, I'm sorry about earlier,' I said.

He nodded.

'Shall we sit?' he replied, scanning my face expectantly. 'Would you like to eat something?'

I shook my head. 'Not enough time.' I glanced at his beautiful face, his pale, soft skin, growing increasingly aware of the intensity of my feelings towards him. 'About earlier, I didn't mean to act like that. I've just got . . . so much going on.'

His shoulders relaxed and he smiled. 'I understand.'

I leaned over the table and took his hand. I watched how the lines on his face smoothed and relaxed as I stroked my thumb over his knuckles. 'I'm in a bit of a hurry, but I was hoping you might take me downstairs. Just for a few minutes,' I said.

'You mean . . . in the mortuary?'

I nodded. 'I want to say goodbye to a former patient of mine.'

I needed to see Dev, to experience some sort of closure, so I could concentrate on moving forward.

Nikolaus released a breath. 'I see! Of course.' He appeared relieved.

'I hope you don't mind me asking.'

'No, I completely understand. I was feeling ashamed for you to know I was working there,' he said. 'It is uncomfortable – and unpleasant, for some people to know I work . . . with dead people.'

I pulled his hand towards me. 'We'll all end up in there, eventually. I'm okay with it.'

'You know, my job there is only temporary, Nina. Where I live, there is a man who has a garage. I rent a room from him. He fixes cars and makes good money. I will do that in the future. I am good at it.'

I nodded. 'It's good to have a plan, Nikolaus. Good to have other skills to rely on.'

We got up and walked towards the lift, Nikolaus carrying a bottle of water under his arm, nibbling a cheese roll he'd bought in the canteen on the way out. Our hands touched and then our fingers knotted more tightly. 'You are talking about the man in the ward, when we saw each other the first time?'

I nodded.

'I remember it now, a terrible situation.'

I closed my eyes, the morphine taking full effect, slowing me down, but my heart beating faster with it.

He pulled his hand away, punching the button for the lower-ground level. The chains rattled and clinked overhead. 'I really appreciate this,' I said. 'I'm sorry to rush you but it's important.'

'Of course,' he said. 'Do as you want. There is no one there at this time of night.'

We entered the double doors leading to the mortuary. Nikolaus keyed in a code and the doors opened.

'Do you like your new job?' I asked.

'I like the quiet,' he said, walking. 'It suits my mind. Although sometimes, when I am alone, I hear noises.'

I stopped suddenly. I wasn't sure whether I'd heard him right. 'What did you say?'

'Noises.'

'What noises?'

'Sometimes they knock from inside the freezer. We do not open the door, however.'

I blinked.

He smiled, then burst out laughing.

I slapped him on the arm.

'That is not funny, Nikolaus. It's almost Halloween. Stuff like that is scary.' But then I laughed too when I saw his eyes sparkling, face stretching into a mischievous smile. I couldn't stop laughing.

'I love to see your happiness,' he said. For a moment, we stared at one another, losing all sense of urgency.

Inside the mortuary, there was a stench of meat, something in between fresh and rotten, mingled with a strange smell of metal. I was struck by how everything around me was beige. The walls, the floors, the fridge doors.

‘How many of you work here?’ I asked. I felt a shiver run down my spine. I glanced around, increasingly uneasy. I couldn’t shake off the feeling that someone was watching us.

‘Five in total, but for a shift, only two. I am taking many shifts so I can save money to buy a good vehicle.’

I glanced at the rows of letter-box drawers, around fifty centimetres high. I wondered how easy it was to slide in like those patients who had prematurely expired.

‘A German car, it must Volkswagen,’ he continued. ‘The build quality is the best.’

I imagined their bodies laid out, waxy and cold, now stiff with rigor mortis. The front desk in the mortuary was piled high with papers. The window to the left was small and barricaded. Above us, the strip lighting flickered. I counted half a dozen dead flies dotting the inside cover.

‘Would you like some tea?’ asked Nikolaus. ‘I have many varieties. English breakfast, of course. But also, herbal.’

I shook my head. ‘I really don’t have time.’ How anyone could think to consume food or drink in this place was bizarre.

I glanced at a roll of black refuse sacks hooked to the wall, a bin in the corner overflowing with Indian takeaway boxes.

I stepped closer to examine a chart:

*Body Fridge Status:*
Bodies for claim x 2
Unclaimed bodies x 8
Coroner cases x 4
HIV x 1

Unclaimed body parts for cremation x 10
Body parts for insurance claims x 5
Muslim body parts x 12
Anything else – unspecified.

'It is the same system for everyone,' said Nikolaus approaching, his voice, his breath, close to my ear. 'No matter who you are or where you come from, it is the same end destination.'

I glanced down.

It was a profound thought. Birth and death entailed so much paperwork, the only two events beyond our control, yet inevitable.

'I wasn't there to prepare Dev's body,' I whispered. 'I feel bad about that. I just couldn't do it.'

I'd prepared bodies before, washing them down shortly after their last exhale. Wrapping them inside a shroud. But I had failed that night, when Dev died.

Nikolaus nodded. 'It is not your fault. Please do not blame yourself. Your boss, Barbara, came from Nightingale to complete the task for you.'

'She did?'

'Of course. It is her job to help.'

I walked to the fridge, utterly deflated that Barbara had stepped in. But that was Barbara for you. No emotion. Clinical. Ready to get the job done with minimal fuss.

I studied the names, handwritten in blue felt-tip pen, stuck to the front doors. There were names of people I didn't know, but in that moment, people I had an overwhelming desire to talk to.

Nikolaus pointed to the door bearing Dev's name.

'He is here, if you want to see him.'

My heart tremored inside my chest.

I walked over to Dev with an overwhelming sense of failure. As nurses, we are trained to look, listen, and feel. To observe changes to breathing, the sound, rhythm, and movement. That night, I had failed to observe. That night, I had been too distracted. 'Do you know what he said to me before he died?' I asked.

Nikolaus was silent.

'That he knew we liked each other . . .'

He placed his hand on my shoulder, then brushed a finger all the way down my arm.

I gave the handle of the beige door a tug. Nikolas stepped back as Dev slid out. I felt the cold prickle my skin as I moved closer to peer at his face. Seeing him like that, lifeless and stiff, covered from the neck down in a white shroud, didn't match the warm, living memory I had of him. I couldn't take my eyes off his face, his eyes peacefully closed. That was when I noticed the strange blotches of blue across his cheekbones.

'What is it?' Nikolaus said, stepping closer.

'His skin. He didn't have those marks before.' My mind searched for something I might have missed.

'After death, the skin can change.'

Nikolaus was right, but Dev had patches of blue on his cheeks, discolouring around his lips.

I lifted the shroud. There were signs of a rash and some mottling on his torso – his chest, arms, lower abdomen. The rash could have been caused by so many factors, from a virus to lupus, low platelets, vasculitis, blood clots, aortic aneurysms – even a reaction to the medication we'd given him. The list was endless.

I glanced up at the clock. I had another seven minutes.

'Can I open his mouth a little? I need to see his tongue.'

Nikolaus swallowed. 'Okay.'

He moved to the side and fetched a pair of plastic gloves as I drifted to the sink to wash my hands. Returning, I took the gloves and snapped them on. I placed my fingers into Dev's mouth. His mouth was dry and cold. I peered inside the cavern and saw his leathery tongue. 'It's very grey.'

My heart began beating faster.

'It is very common, I am sure of it,' said Nikolaus.

'I'd better go,' I said after a while, my arm dropping. 'It's getting late, and this is . . . unhelpful. He's gone. What more can I do . . .' I mumbled to myself.

'You are sure?'

I nodded. I was not even sure what I was looking for with an investigation already underway.

I slid Dev back into the fridge, peeled off my gloves and washed my hands once more with soap.

I turned, drying my hands; Nikolaus glanced down. We walked to the door and he paused before fully opening it.

'There is a back entrance that leads to the main road, up the ramp. It is where the vans and other vehicles come for funerals. There is also a café at the top. Maybe we have some breakfast . . . when you have more time.'

'I'd love that.' I smiled. 'Or you could just come to mine . . .' I reached for his hand.

He moved his body, his face, closer to mine. 'Maybe it's better. My room smells of oil and petrol.'

I laughed, closing my eyes, ready for him to take me whenever and however he wanted.

We heard a clang in one of the fridges.

I jolted. 'What the hell is that?'

Nikolaus laughed.

'See? I told you: they try to escape . . .'

# 16

The following afternoon, I took it slow. Every move was careful and controlled. I was thinking things over as I lay in bed, a slip of sunlight warming my face. I realised how much effort I'd put in the wrong places. All this time, my life had been about work, work, work, nothing about *me*. I hadn't properly taken care of my mental health, nor any of my relationships.

I stared at the leaflet they gave me at work, now pinned to the corkboard on the wall. The Royal College of Nursing ran a nurses' counselling service. I made myself a cup of tea and thought it was high time I changed things.

I dialled the number at the bottom and waited for someone to pick up.

'Hello. Nurses' Careline. How can we help?'

'I think I need to talk to someone,' I said.

'Is it the counselling service you need, or the legal helpline?'

I needed both, but I thought it was best to stick with counselling. I knew I needed to talk about what happened with Dev, how I'd let it all get on top of me these past few days. Besides, with an investigation in motion, it would be beneficial to inform them at work I'd done it. I'd sought help. That conversation I'd overheard in the toilets between Barbara and Sandra still infuriated me.

A woman called Amy noted my details and promised to pass them on to the next available therapist.

'Frances is available. She's good – inundated with requests, though. She's free for online sessions if that's at all useful?' Amy's voice was chirpy. 'You should receive a Zoom link this evening. If your availability changes, just send us an email.'

After I hung up, I opened Safari and searched for Leroy Sanchez. I wanted to see whether he lived online, learn a little about his identity and life. He'd ruined mine and taken Dev's. The least I was owed were a few essential details.

The search revealed hundreds of entries for a Spanish singer-songwriter, first discovered on YouTube. But nothing for the criminal of Newgate who had stabbed Balraj. It was odd that a man like that had no online presence. He was a digital ghost, no mention of him anywhere.

I searched Google Images. Videos. News. Still, nothing.

Next, I scrolled through Google reviews of Newgate Hospital as if wanting, perversely, to punish myself by reinforcing just how awful it really was.

Mehta.1.2.3
*Newgate is a joke. I was in agony with a potential toe fracture, but instead of helping me, I waited six hours!*

Christina Pardesi_1487
*I don't care how stressed or stretched they are, nurses should not shout at patients. I have never come across such rude nurses as the ones employed at Newgate. I can understand now why this hospital has been sued so many times for negligence.*

NHS_Whistle_Blower

*It's sad when you see an NHS hospital getting a 1-star rating, but honestly, it deserves nothing more. Staff are rude, incompetent and don't communicate with you properly. You end up feeling exploited by the state because there is no alternative available. It's like they are ruining it on purpose but still charging taxes.*

Nigel_Watkins

*Too many of them are foreign and don't speak good enough English. And these days, there's so many police in A&E. It's like being in an episode of a crime series!*

That evening, I clicked on the Zoom link I'd received from Amy. I waited as the screen loaded, and two black boxes appeared. I saw myself in the box on the left, and then, after a short while, Frances appeared on the right. She was seated against an elegant home-office background – a tall bay window, a chesterfield leather sofa, two leafy rubber plants.

'Nice to meet you, Nina.'

She appeared thin and frail, wearing a white cardigan, an oversized silver clip in her hair. Her face was pale and make-up free. Her voice, steely and centred.

'Hello,' I said.

I placed my laptop on the coffee table, shuffling the newspapers and takeaway flyers into a pile. 'I appreciate the time you're giving me.'

'Not at all. It's all part of your membership. Shall we start with you talking a little bit about yourself?'

I explained to Frances that I was a nurse in charge at Newgate Hospital, qualified in the summer of 2017. We discussed how, like most nurses, I'd been thrown into the pandemic with little warning. I was hoping the internet didn't lag because I didn't want to have to repeat all that.

'You're not alone. So many nurses have been struggling ever since COVID. It's important you know that. Also, that you don't feel ashamed because you're seeking emotional assistance.'

That made me feel more at ease, but not enough to tell Frances about the tablets, nor how close I'd been to stabbing Leroy with scissors. But then, there was Dev. I did need to get the weight of that terrible night off my chest.

'Is there anyone else you're currently talking to or is this your first session?'

'I do have a friend, but conversations like this are a bit different.' I thought of Mercedes, so strong and together. The last thing she needed was for me to be a burden.

Frances scribbled something down. 'So, what happened?'

I told her what happened. That I had no choice but to prioritise Leroy that night, and the consequences.

'And how do you feel now?'

'Numb. A bit spaced out. Dissociated from myself, which is a blessing, considering what's going on. I can't stop blaming myself, but also, I don't think it's fair. There's no way nurses can be *everywhere*.'

'I understand how you feel, but it's not your fault,' she said.

She was right, it wasn't me. I blamed Leroy and now I wanted him dead. *He* should have died that night.

Frances began typing.

'Are you taking any medication to help you through this?'

The tablets didn't count. That was private. 'No, nothing.'

More typing: the tap-tap of fingernails made my teeth feel funny.

'It might be helpful to know that there is nothing wrong with you,' said Frances.

*That's a relief.*

'That everything you're describing is perfectly natural given the circumstances. You need time to process what's happened. It's tough now, but in time, it will make you stronger. Every nurse goes through it.'

I was about to say thank you, that was just what I needed to hear, but could we go a bit deeper because I had these dark feelings I needed to explore. But just like that, Frances froze on screen. Her mouth wide open, eyes firmly closed. I almost wanted to laugh at the comedy of it all. But I felt the urge to burst into tears, also.

A message popped up in the chat.

*Sorry! My connection has dropped. I can't see or hear you. Are you still there?*

I couldn't help but wonder why anyone thought Zoom therapy was a good idea. Before I could answer my own question, a longer message appeared.

*The RCN has some great free resources to help you with potential symptoms of trauma. Have you been on their website?*

I typed a message back.

*I am a member, so yes, I've seen their stuff.*

*Great! You can stick with this counselling service, but they won't support you longer term if you're already receiving support elsewhere. Otherwise, you're doubling up.*

*Can I stick with you?* I wrote.

*Of course:-) What's your number? Maybe it's better if I call you?*

Within seconds, Frances was on the phone apologising. Although I couldn't see her, I did feel something shifting. Her voice was wonderfully calm and having a positive effect on me.

'I think maybe I need more opportunities to talk about it,' I said. 'Perhaps I don't talk about things enough. Maybe there are a few techniques I could integrate with more sessions. I'd be open to it.'

Frances rattled off a list, which I suspected she had in front of her.

'So, the first is to take more care of yourself, particularly during this difficult time. Remember the three Rs: Rest, Rehydrate and Refuel. Taking regular breaks and exercise is vital.'

'That's not always easy,' I said.

'You can insist,' she said. 'Second . . .' She took a sip of something to drink. I heard her swallow and smack her lips.

'There's a good range of well-being apps packed with information where you can record your feelings and keep track of your emotions.'

'Like a menstruation app?'

Frances hesitated. 'I suppose you could say that. That's in addition to talking therapy, which will help.'

But I wasn't keen. The last app I'd downloaded was an app for yoga, which cost me £7.99 a month, and which I couldn't afford to keep paying.

'Finally, I recommend you start jotting down your feelings in a reflective journal. Daily journaling has huge benefits. It helps establish new neural pathways, keeping you sharp and agile. It will help you process what's happened.'

I was silent.

'Reflecting on our experiences is a universal need. Writing things down helps us process unconscious feelings.'

'But what if I find writing hard?' I said. The truth is, I was not very good at it. Ever since I could remember, I had been a terrible student.

'You don't need to write in complete sentences. Half sentences or keywords – that's already tremendous.'

I thought I was in the wrong job, because compared to nursing, therapy was straightforward.

'Thank you,' I said. 'I'm ever so grateful.'

Frances hung up.

I realised I still had the phone in my hand and was listening to dead air.

I'd spent most of my life being grateful. Maybe there lay the root of all my problems. I was *grateful* I was found in the phone box that day. *Grateful* that although I'd been placed in a foster home, made to complete all household chores with my own bare hands, including changing the nappies of angry toddlers, I did not endure any other form of abuse like most of the other kids did. I was *grateful* I'd got out, that I'd ended up in Maple Tree where I'd met Mercedes. *Grateful* for the financial assistance I'd received from charities to train as a nurse. *Grateful* to Balraj for discounting my rent. *Grateful* I'd got my first placement in a hospital like Newgate. *Grateful* to have a job, even when it entailed people threatening violence, doling out racist abuse, soiling sheets, spitting coffee in my face on the very best of occasions.

'Thank you,' I said, the dead air filling my ears.

But as I put the phone down, I'd decided: there would be no more giving thanks.

# 17

On my way to work the following night, I couldn't shake the feeling that I was being followed.

I saw a white VW Polo, muddy smear to the side, pass my flat when I left home. And then from the back of the moving bus, I saw it again, overtaking us. By the time I reached the hospital car park, the same car was parked between a blue Hyundai i30 and a silver Toyota Camry.

The sky was dirty grey, the rain fell hard. I wondered what would happen when I got into work. Whether the mandatory investigation into Dev's death had concluded, whether I'd lost my job.

Even though nursing didn't pay much, barely enough to live on, the thought of having no income at all was far worse. If they cited negligence or found I'd been stealing medication, I'd be permanently struck off. One word with Ravi was all it would take. I'd never be able to practise nursing again.

In the canteen, I found a seat in the furthest corner beside the window and sat down with my coffee. After a few minutes, Farah walked in. She nodded at me, strangely, as if knowing I'd be there. She ordered herself a drink and I swallowed hard as it occurred to me that it was her all along, following me.

She sauntered over with a mug in her hand.

'Mind if I join you?' Not really a request.

I nodded. 'I wasn't expecting to see you here.'

'Like to keep people on their toes. Besides, hardly anyone's around this time of night. Has its advantages.'

I noted she didn't look me in the eye.

'I was here to see Balraj as well.' She sat down, removing the teabag from her mug. 'Didn't startle you, did I?'

'Have you been following me?' I asked.

She stared at me and scoffed, but didn't answer.

'How is Balraj?' I asked.

She leaned back and sighed. 'Oh, you know. Holding up, given the circumstances. But he's not walking. Most likely, he never will. But I figure you probably know that already.'

I looked around me. The canteen was empty, which was a relief. It was really not a good idea to be seen talking to a journalist. 'I did hear. Look . . . are you wanting to check whether I've managed to, y'know, get anything on Newgate?' I leaned in closer. 'Because I haven't – not yet. But I *will*. There's definitely something going on. It's just better if I talk to you outside . . .'

Farah took a sip of her tea.

'Here's a bit *public*, and I'm supposed to be starting a shift,' I said.

'Nina,' she said, her voice lowered. 'I need to talk to you about Dev.'

I felt the blood drain from my face. *Sandra. That bitch, that fucking cow. What has she said?*

'I need to go,' I said. I got up to leave, rushing towards the door, but Farah followed behind me.

'Nina, I just want to hear *your* version, that's all!'

In the corridor, I walked as quickly as I could, but Farah easily caught up, gathering speed until she was trotting to the side of me. 'I imagine you can't be happy about what's going on in the hospital. But now, see, there are complaints about *you*. Anything you want to say before I write up the story and draw my own conclusions?'

I stopped dead in my tracks as two doctors rushed past. 'Sorry, what?'

'You made errors, I heard. Put Dev at risk. That's not what we want in hospitals, now, is it?'

I stared at this woman, who, for a second, I imagined would be exactly the sort I'd have given a good kicking to at school. One minute your friend, another quick to knife you in the stomach. 'You've been following me – for this?'

'Not exactly.' She shuffled her feet. 'I've been wanting to talk to you more generally.'

I walked off again, my heart pounding, mind racing. Wanting to get the hell out of there and straight into Florence Nightingale. I was walking so fast, she struggled to keep up.

'So, you think it's unfair? That they shouldn't implicate you?' Farah said.

'What are you talking about?' I stopped once more. 'There's a mandatory inquiry going on. They've not communicated findings yet,' I said, panting.

'Look,' Farah spoke quickly, quietly. 'The mother . . . she came to see me. Something is fishy, Nina. Your name was mentioned. I must tell you that your version most likely contradicts hers.'

'What are you saying, exactly?'

'Everything points to negligence. But from where I'm standing, it's incompetence that's causing the problems. It's hard to overlook what's happening on the ground.'

It was all I needed. A social warrior, trying to make a name out of the local news, so that she could get herself a job at the *Guardian*.

I laughed. 'You've got this all wrong.'

'This is the story I have.'

I slipped past Farah, walking, then running faster.

Farah grabbed my arm. 'Give me something more if you have it,' she said.

'I'll find something,' I replied. 'I *told* you: I'm working on it. Believe me, what I have for you is a story far bigger than this. This isn't the story you want . . . nurses falling victim to stretched resources. The real story is about vested interests with disastrous consequences for this hospital – for the community of Levinstone.'

'Vested interests,' Farah said, her voice clipped.

'I'm working on gathering information. It will be big.' I stared at her without blinking. It was a lie, of course, a complete lie. I had nothing concrete. But what choice did I have?

Farah looked down, thinking. 'I'm filing a story this week. If you don't give me another story, I'll have no choice but to write *this* one. I'm under pressure too. Local stories like this are powerful.'

*Fucking journalists.* Now I knew why everyone hated them.

'I told you, I have something, but I need time to gather evidence. Don't trash me in the papers based on a grieving mother's account. You don't know the half of it. Some of us need to make a living. We don't have rich parents. We've come from nothing. You understand that, don't you? It will ruin my life, and I've done nothing wrong.' I bit my lip.

'I'll give you until the end of the week.' Farah's tone hardened. 'Again, here's my number.' She gave me her card and walked off towards the main entrance.

The doors whooshed open; I pressed my back against the wall. I stared down at the card, my fingers brushing over the letters, F-A-R-A-H . . .

I walked into Florence Nightingale, my thoughts swirling, chest tight. I needed to hurry up and find evidence because I wanted Farah out of my life. But then, that smell of the ward brought it up for me again. That sight of Leroy's face pressed in my mind with greater ferocity. He was like a germ, spreading, multiplying, no matter how much I tried to scrub myself clean.

I sent Mercedes a text:

*Need to talk to you ASAP. Where r u???*

Mercedes:
*Was having dinner with S. Having a heart to heart. I need to be paid more for my services!! Why, what's up?? xxx*

Nina:
*72 hours is up soon. I'm getting worried! I need tangible proof that something dodgy is going on in here or we are all screwed! A journalist from the* Gazette *is*

*going to trash me in the press about Dev! Says it's all my fault.*

Mercedes:
*No way! How did she get your name? No wonder they're paranoid about journalists sniffing around. But what evidence does she have but hearsay?? Stay calm. We can chat in the morning. I've got a shift. Did you see the all-staffer?*

In the corridor, I bumped into Preeti. She appeared coy, straining a smile before lowering her eyes.

'Everything okay?' I asked.

She pursed her lips and nodded. But her smile was off. Sandra had most likely poisoned her against me, after all the support I'd offered. And what *was* that look Preeti gave me just now? A frown, a dose of *pity*? On the perspex floor, my legs felt strangely heavy. I watched her turn the corner and considered running after her. But when I glanced left, I caught sight of Leroy in his room. He was standing beside his bed, his back bent, a hand clutching the frame. Barry was beside him, his hand on Leroy's shoulder, like a father might congratulate his son after a well-played football match.

I took a deep breath, reminding myself to stay strong. I was relieved to see Leroy on his feet. It meant he'd likely be discharged – it couldn't have come any sooner. Barry looked up and waved.

'It's like he's getting out of jail.' Barry laughed as I approached him. The joke was so badly timed.

'Yeah, well, I'm glad to be getting out of here,' Leroy

said. He tipped his head in my direction. 'Did I tell you she creeps up on patients in the middle of the night, scaring the shit out of them when they're vulnerable. Fucking weird, it is. She's not normal.' Leroy folded his clothes, neatly placing them into his shabby holdall. Though he moved slowly, carefully, he appeared stronger, almost fully healed.

I ignored his comment and walked further into the room. I found a woman slumped on a chair, scrolling through her phone. I knew that must be Leroy's mother. *Poor woman, to have spent her life justifying why she gave birth to him.* When she looked up, I realised I'd seen that face before.

'We haven't met.' I said, but we had, at the community meeting in the church. I'd listened to Grace drone on about the need for non-judgement.

Grace peered at me as I reached out my hand. She re-arranged her brown cardigan and uncrossed her legs, extending her hand to shake mine.

'Thank you for taking care of my son.' She looked down, retreating to her phone as if engrossed in a text conversation. It was clear she hadn't recognised me.

'I hope you enjoyed your stay,' I said to Leroy, standing with my arms crossed.

'Don't change the subject,' he spat. 'There's something wrong with you. It's dangerous when nurses hold grudges.'

'Come now. I'm just doing my job,' I said.

'Bullshit.'

'Steady on, son,' said Barry. 'She's the nurse that helped you back onto your feet. Was around when your mum could not be here. That's no way to talk to her. You owe her some appreciation, at least.' Barry glanced at me, rolling his eyes.

It was as if to say *What can you do, he's just like a child.*

'Hurry up,' Grace said. 'I've made dinner for us. At least now I can keep an eye on you, and you'll have no choice but to stay indoors.'

'I'm sorry to hear you didn't find our service satisfactory,' I scoffed, moving to the end of the bed, lifting Leroy's notes clamped under the metal claw of the clipboard. 'Only, you hogged enough resources.'

Barry was taken aback. Grace writhed awkwardly in her chair.

'See what I mean?' said Leroy. He held up his hands, pleading with Barry, but then he winced, placing his hand on his stomach. 'She's got a problem.' He turned to his mother. 'Mum! Do you see it?'

Grace shook her head, throwing me a stormy glare. 'Pack your bags, son. We need to get out of here.' She stood up. 'Do we have a problem here?'

'Maybe ask your son. A real pillar of the community, it seems.'

I snorted as Grace was taken aback.

'If you're antagonising him, in his condition, I'll have you reported.'

'Entirely your decision,' I said. 'Though it's unlikely to make much difference.' But in that moment, something clicked. I realised I was getting myself into serious trouble when I was already in a vulnerable position.

There was a knock on the door, and I looked up from the notes.

Barbara appeared in the doorway. 'Nina, do you have a minute?' Her grey hair was haloed in light. I caught a glimpse of Sandra scuttling past, just behind her. 'Won't take long.'

I lowered my head quickly, feigning casual. 'Of course.'

I left Barry to help Leroy pack up the last of his things: a razor, grubby towel, a stack of books on social justice. I wondered how Grace, as his mother, could just sit there, so relaxed. Was Leroy Barry's illegitimate child? Certainly, he behaved as though he was.

As I walked behind Barbara, threading through the stuffy corridor, I wondered how much of my exchange with Leroy she'd heard. Barbara's scrubs were stiff, starch pressed, her curls compact. I caught a whiff of her lavender scent. It reminded me of an old-fashioned era, a quintessentially English vibe.

She nodded as we turned to the right. 'In here,' she said.

I sat down in her office. Barbara moved to the window, staring out into the car park below.

'What on earth was that tone just now? I didn't catch it all, but what I did catch did not sound good.'

'That was a criminal, who crippled a man,' I said. 'He's receiving the very best treatment in the NHS, courtesy of hard-working taxpayers.'

Barbara shook her head. 'Twenty years. That's how long I've been doing this,' she said.

I glanced down at the floor.

'I've seen it all. Births, sudden deaths. Assaults on nurses – all manner of emergencies.'

I wasn't sure where this was going.

'In a strange way, I sympathise with your views. But they have no place in the NHS. You know that, don't you?'

I pinched the skin on my hands, reminding myself that, no matter how much my thoughts flitted and scampered, I had better pay close attention.

'This job is hard, Nina. You don't need to make it harder for yourself, nor the rest of us.'

I could hardly disagree. I wondered whether I should tell Barbara I was doing a few counselling sessions to help me better cope with things.

'Why am I here?' I asked.

Barbara sighed, glancing down.

'I know you took Dev's death hard,' she said. 'There's always one that cuts deep. I also know you did your best, but you should know . . .'

I felt my eyes well.

'We've had the coroner's report back along with the results of the mandatory seventy-two-hour investigation.'

I swallowed hard.

'There are some discrepancies that have raised serious questions.'

'Like what exactly?' I said hurriedly. 'Can you at least give me some idea?'

She drew a deep breath. 'I probably shouldn't say this, but between you and me, the main issue is that the morphine prescribed by Dr Milburn was not recorded in the notes and is missing from Dev's medication chart.'

A wave of panic gripped me.

'Dev did not have morphine in his system, either – which is strange. The coroner has confirmed this, but Dr Milburn is certain he prescribed it. I've said too much. Maria should explain all this. But what it means is that we need to continue investigating, to ascertain what really happened. This, plus other omissions in the notes – no mention of the hydrocortisone cream you applied to his rash, plus concerns regarding your general attitude and tone as I witnessed just now. It's enough to . . .' Barbara clenched her jaw.

'It was Manisha – the mother,' I said. '*She* was against him taking morphine after theatre. That's why it's not in his system. Sure, I possibly forgot to record the hydrocortisone cream. It was an innocent mistake.'

'The second dose of morphine prescribed, too?'

'Excuse me?'

'You say the mother advised her son not to take the dose prescribed after theatre. But what about the second dose of morphine prescribed by Dr Milburn – when Dev was on the ward and in pain?'

'I believe the mother refused those too.' My face burned. I felt ashamed to lie. But there was no way I could tell them what I did that night. They'd report me to the NMC. 'She didn't want him taking morphine in the absence of a firm diagnosis. It was perfectly understandable.'

'But it was not recorded in Dev's medication chart, and morphine was not found in Dev's system. The tablets are missing. We've spoken to Manisha. She was not aware of a second prescription.'

I dropped my head.

'It's not just the morphine, is it? That's bad enough, but Nina, what did I witness just now, hmm? With Leroy?' She sounded like a schoolteacher.

'I can explain—'

But at that moment, Maria Gonzalez walked in. I tried

so hard to avoid her eyes, but she caught mine.

'Just in time,' said Barbara to Maria. Barbara cleared her throat and turned to me, cold and formal. 'As you know, Maria has been overseeing the investigation. We want to avoid speculation until we've clarified precise details.'

Maria sat down in the corner, her oud perfume pungent, and also the smell of cheese and onion.

Barbara shrugged her shoulders. 'You need to understand, you were the nurse on duty. Dev was in your care. If there are discrepancies, we must continue an investigation.'

I noticed how Barbara's face dropped, how she looked straight at me.

'What did he die from?' I asked, my voice low.

'Sudden cardiac death, during his sleep.'

I felt my throat quiver.

'But there's so much more to it that we need to explore. We can't go into details,' said Maria.

'Can't or won't?' I asked.

'Just like we won't go into the details of your behaviour with Leroy and his mother, just now,' said Barbara. 'But you must understand, I'm obliged to log it as all part of this investigation's findings. It will form part of the final report.'

'This meeting is about particular discrepancies,' chipped Maria. 'Inaccurate recording keeping – that is, failure to mention that you'd applied hydrocortisone cream topically to a rash and given Dev a Piriton tablet on the evening of 21st October at approximately 10 p.m. when Dr Milburn had seen him. That early sign could have been significant.'

*Significant?*

She was not wrong. I saw a flash of Dev in the mortuary. The patches of blue smeared across his cheekbones.

'Mainly, it's about the morphine,' she said, 'prescribed but not administered, and still missing. It's led us to make further enquiries. We know you had a conversation with Ravi. But you failed to mention it to Barbara.' Maria paused. 'There's plenty here and it's serious.'

I clenched my jaw.

'You can't deny you've not been yourself,' Barbara said. 'I've been observing you closely. You've been distracted, brusque with patients. I know how hard you've worked. I know how stressed you've been. But many nurses have stated you've been unnecessarily harsh. Today I witnessed it.'

'If you're unable to offer indiscriminate care, you can't be a nurse. It's that simple,' Maria said, shaking her head. 'You know the Code.'

Of course I did. I knew it by heart. But now it meant nothing.

'This is all being kept internal for now,' offered Barbara. 'I appreciate it's a lot to take in. Currently, we're treating this as an employment matter rather than something logged with the NMC. But we need to suspend you with immediate effect, while we continue our investigation.'

'To clarify, you'll receive full pay,' said Maria, almost cheerful.

My eyes scanned the room and I felt them fill. Teardrops fell into my lap and bled into the blue material. Of course, I knew I was in the wrong. I had stolen morphine, and of all the points mentioned, this was the most serious. But in the grand scheme of things, it did not seem fair. An absence of morphine could not be the cause of Dev's death.

'I tried to help Dev, but we were overstretched. There's no way we could cope with the number of admissions.'

'Our focus is on your work, not the issues of wider healthcare provision,' said Maria.

I wanted to slap her, really, I did.

'I need to remind you that you are prohibited from speaking to the press. I appreciate this might feel like a shock.' Barbara moved to the water cooler, pulling a plastic glass from the side. She pressed the nozzle to dispense water and handed me a glass. 'Drink. Keep yourself hydrated. Last thing we need is for you to get sick at this important moment.'

My hands trembled as I held on to the cup. I wished it was something stronger because I felt like they were stitching me up. They blamed me for Dev's death. It had nothing to do with the morphine. And, just now with Leroy, who could blame me?

'I need a minute,' I said, 'to get my things.'

'Of course,' said Barbara. 'Do what you need to and go gently. Come back tomorrow morning if you need more time. But after that, you need to hand in your pass. I'll email you in a few days.'

Maria stood up, straightening her jacket. She nodded to Barbara. 'We'll be in touch,' she said.

That evening in the canteen, wearing an old blue tracksuit, I snatched glances at the other nurses, mainly women, who'd been my support network all these years. They appeared strangely distant, like they knew what was going on. Seated at the table eating my cheese roll, I watched Preeti and Sandra move to the front, helping themselves to tea and coffee. Preeti lifted the plastic lid of the pastry box and took out a doughnut. She was absorbed in conversation, shaking her head, talking to Sandra as if unable to believe that a certain something had *actually* happened. Sandra shrugged her shoulders in a statement that appeared to confirm, perhaps, it was inevitable. The signs were there from the start.

They might not have been talking about me. I might just have been paranoid.

I fired Mercedes a text, asking her to meet me urgently because everything felt like it was collapsing.

*Are you awake?? I did something stupid, M. They're blaming me for what happened to Dev. I was not responsible – I swear!!! Call me. xxx*

Mercedes replied:

*I know. They're saying you were negligent. Something about morphine stolen, but I know it's lies. They are all bastards. I told you, didn't I? Don't talk to ANYONE. There's already too much gossiping going on in Newgate! We WILL straighten this out! I promise. Let's meet tomorrow.*

I pulled out my wallet from my bag and opened it up. I spotted Farah's card and prised it out. I may not be perfect, and for sure, I'd seriously fucked up. But there was no way I was going down for this.

# 18

The next morning, I headed towards the hospital car park and waited at the back, leaning a shoulder against a graffitied wall beside a giant recycling container. I glanced at my phone and felt a tap on my shoulder.

Mercedes smiled and grabbed my arm. We moved to hug one another, and I felt my body relax.

'How are you holding up?' she asked as I pulled away.

'It hasn't fully hit me yet . . .'

She placed an arm around my shoulder, moving me further to the side. We stood under a grey awning outside, thin threads of light weaving onto the tarmac. 'Did you collect your stuff, or do you need me to get anything for you?'

'I've got it,' I said, tapping my bag. 'I'm about to give them my card. I need to get out of this place as soon as I can.'

'Bastards,' mumbled Mercedes.

'They're still paying me, at least.'

'It's not about money, though, is it? Anyway, it's like you said, lots of people have stories to tell – especially that journalist, Farah. I hear she's been sniffing around. Did you read the all-staff email? They're being extra careful.'

I stared at Mercedes. 'Do you know her?'

'No.' She shifted the weight between her feet. 'You mentioned her name.'

'I did?'

'Yeah, you did.'

Mercedes glanced to the side.

'Well, yeah, I imagine she's hunting for a story on Newgate, and if she doesn't get one, she'll focus on cases of negligence,' I said. 'Nurses on the front line, just trying to do their jobs like everyone else.'

Mercedes bit her lip. 'What are you thinking?'

'I'm thinking I should give her a story. The new supplier framework – the insane number of tests we had to carry out on Dev. Something's going on. Remember what Mary said. Richard has conflicts of interest. What if it's true?' I leaned back on the wall, trying to find a comfortable spot for my back to sink into the brickwork. 'We need to get to the bottom of all this somehow and expose them.'

Mercedes stared hard, then rummaged in her pocket for her cigarette packet. She lit one up, her fingers trembling. 'How will you gather the information you need, exactly?'

I straightened. 'Well, for starters, I need to establish if there's a link between Richard and MediCentral. We all know he pushed them through to deliver off-site testing. No one wanted it. There's bound to be something to prove the rumours. Relationships are traceable. Having a vested interest would explain why he's so keen to integrate them into service pathways.'

'Evidence like that will be hard to find,' said Mercedes. 'He would have been careful not to leave a paper trail.'

'There's always a paper trail,' I said. 'It would also be good to get numbers on how many tests have been carried out versus patients admitted – to chart if that number has spiked suspiciously. And I need a chat with the lab staff to see if they know anything. But that is sensitive. They might not talk.'

Mercedes was thinking. 'You can't do this alone. You need helpers. Presumably the idea is that you then send all this to Farah. Get her to stop sniffing around if she's got what she needs?'

I really didn't know Farah too well. It occurred to me how little information I had concerning her background. I made a mental note to use my newly found free time to look her up. 'A journalist like Farah will know what to do with information like that,' I said.

Mercedes flicked ash onto the ground. 'I bet Sunil and Reggie might help. That would get you IT access and keys to the management office, but God, that is risky.'

I stared into the distance. 'I don't have much choice, do I?'

We watched as a family of four entered their car, a man climbing into the driver's seat. We stood, the two of us in silence, my bag weighing heavily on my shoulder.

'I shouldn't be telling you this,' I said. 'I don't want to get you into trouble, or to risk you losing your job. It's bad enough that I'm in this position. Just forget I mentioned it.'

She looked down, her brow twitching. 'I have a bad feeling about all this. But I know you won't listen.'

She threw down her cigarette and moved closer and I gave her a hug.

'Watch your back, Nina,' she said. 'And whatever you do, don't trust anyone.'

I pulled away and nodded.

It was a conflict, all this. I knew I had no choice, but I also knew it would not be easy. I felt torn, too, bringing the profession I loved into disrepute. Nursing was ingrained into my muscle memory. Caring for others was an instinct. I didn't want to destroy the hospital when I'd loved working there. But that thought of Leroy, laughing at me, telling me I was mad. *Oi, you, nurse. You're a psycho, do you know that?*

And then there was Balraj, an innocent member of our community, lying in a hospital bed and now paralysed. Leroy distracted me that night, unleashing in me the worst possible kind of person.

'I'll be fine,' I said. 'I just appreciate you listening. That's already helpful.' My eyes filled; my voice broke. 'I'd better go,' I said.

Mercedes smiled.

'There's just one last thing I need to do on my way out.'

In the Lighthouse Tower, I stood beside Balraj's bed, watching his eyes twitch, then open, as he sensed my presence.

'Nina . . .' He licked his lips, struggling to smile. He moved his fingers a little.

I reached out my hand, resting it on his shoulder as I fought back the tears. 'I came to see how you're feeling, but you mustn't strain yourself.'

He swallowed.

'I will leave Levinstone . . . it is no more for me.'

I pulled a chair closer and sat down. 'You don't mean that, Balraj. This is your home. What you're going through, the pain, the anguish, *will* pass, I promise. I believe in karma. I believe in justice.' But I was unsure whether I truly did.

I placed my hand upon his, feeling him warm, but also weak.

He was silent, breathing hard. 'I give myself time to recover . . . but Sheela is not so happy, now.'

I closed my eyes, attempting to ingest his words, to push them down deep where all my disappointment lurked. The beep-beep-beep of the heart monitor made me sit up. I scanned Balraj's arms still stickered with dressings. His grazes and bruises were healing, but the damage left was irreversible.

'I am tired . . . I realise how tired I am, lying here,' he said.

I was tired too, so tired. I wanted out.

I watched his eyes close, his chest relax. I drew the curtains around him to allow his breath to better settle.

# 19

Halloween. A knock on the door. For a split second, I forgot where I was. Lying in bed between the blur of dreaming and wakefulness, I pictured myself still on the ward. I thought I'd fallen asleep on the sofa in the staffroom still wearing full scrubs. Panic gripped me like the arm cuff on a blood pressure monitoring machine. I was certain I'd missed the other nurses calling out to me.

But I was at home. I drew a deep breath and hauled myself up. I told myself that, no matter what, I'd soldier on. That's what a good nurse does.

The knock came again. Through the peephole I saw Nikolaus at the top of the stairwell.

I rushed to the mirror, frantically brushing my hair, spraying perfume onto my neck.

Nikolaus was about to leave as I turned the handle.

He blushed, seeing me standing there in my robe.

'Hi,' he said, holding out a bunch of flowers. He was clean-shaven; the silver zips on his leather jacket sparkled.

'I wasn't expecting you,' I said.

'I heard what happened. I was worried.'

My mouth was dry.

I took the flowers, pressing my nose into the soft petals, the heaviness of the morning and early afternoon lifting a little. 'They're beautiful,' I said. 'Nobody has ever bought me flowers before.'

He smiled as I opened the door wider to let him in. He glanced around as if remembering, with some fondness, the last time we were both here.

'What did you hear exactly?' I closed the door, moving to the kitchen sink to place the flowers on the counter.

'That you were staying at home because of the investigation.'

I nodded. He didn't run; that was a relief. 'Would you like some tea?' I urged him to take a seat.

We sat together at the kitchen table for a while, sipping from our mugs. I told him everything that had happened.

'It is not your fault. You did your best.' Nikolaus placed his hand upon mine. 'I do not know you very well, but in my heart, I know this much.'

I stared into his eyes, moved that he trusted and accepted me as I was. I felt vulnerable yet safe in his presence, assured he would never let me down. And yet, deep inside, I felt an uncertainty, too. There was a little voice in my head telling me not to trust him nor to give in to him too easily. Everyone in my life always let me down.

We moved to the sofa and he drew nearer. We lay on our sides, our bodies spooning as one. He nuzzled his face into my neck and wrapped his arms securely across my stomach.

'Sometimes, difficult days come to test us,' he whispered.

I closed my eyes, fighting off that gremlin voice. 'I just feel like I've had so many of them.'

'I do as well,' he said. 'But we have each other, now. That is something special.'

I turned my face; my lips met his. I felt the brush of velvet from his tongue, and I melted.

'Are you working today?' I asked as I pulled away, airy and breathless.

'No.'

'Then let's stay like this all evening.'

I had to learn to trust him, no matter how uncomfortable it was. To think he had appeared now, to carry me through, when so much of my life was uncertain.

The smile on his face told me he needed and wanted me too.

I snuggled close to him, placing my head on his chest. I listened to his heartbeat, felt the wonderful rhythm of his movements.

I wanted to sleep, to feel every tick of his body, to soak in the gentle warmth of him.

'I regret I did not do so well in school,' he said. 'That I must work these manual kinds of jobs to earn money.'

I held on to him ever more tightly.

'I was hardly a good student,' I said.

'But you are a good nurse.'

'And you can read and write – German and English. Most of us here speak only one language.'

He laughed as I placed my head on his stomach, listening to the faint gurgles and bubbles of his organs. 'Are you hungry?' I asked after a while.

'Certainly, I am now,' he said.

I diced then fried an onion in a smear of oil, watching the onions sweat in the pan. Steam rose under the cooking hood, and my eyes watered from the pungent smell. I boiled water, reduced the heat, then threw in dried pasta shells.

I was turning the spatula when Nikolaus drew closer, holding me from behind.

'If you do that, the pasta will overcook and it's all I have to feed you.' I laughed.

He kissed my neck, moving to nibble my ear. 'I am okay with that,' he whispered.

A splash of boiling water from the pan burned my hand. Instinctively, I pushed him back. Dev appeared in my mind, blue-tongued. A flash and flicker of Dr Milburn from that night.

'You are okay?' he said.

'It's nothing.'

Dev was dead. A young man who'd had his whole life ahead of him, who'd told me he had dreams of marrying, was gone. The voice inside my head pressed stronger now. It asked me who I thought I was, being selfish, thinking only of myself. Acting like nothing had happened. But I was *owed* this, wasn't I? I'd waited so long to find a kindred spirit. Never did I imagine he'd turn up at Newgate.

The onions turned golden. I opened a can of chopped tomatoes. Nikolaus was beside the open window, staring out onto the pavement.

'It is getting cold now,' he said.

I snorted as I threw the tomatoes into the pan. 'You're turning into a real Brit, talking about the weather.'

I removed the boiled pasta from the hob, draining the water through a colander. 'Pasta is served,' I said. 'Sorry, no parmesan.'

We settled at the table with a jug of water. Nikolaus devoured his food like he'd never eaten anything so delicious.

'What will you do now you are at home?'

I stared into space. 'Not sure. I'll find something to do, I suppose.'

'You can move – you have a car?'

'I do, but it's out of service. I'll take the bus if I need to. It's easier.'

He stared at me, dabbing his mouth with a paper towel.

'You have a car, but you are preferring to take the bus?'

'Too expensive to fix,' I said. 'Dodgy suspension.'

He placed his fork down.

'Come,' he said, finishing his pasta. 'We will fix it tonight.'

I laughed awkwardly, swallowing tomato sauce. 'Don't be silly. You don't need to do that.'

'Why not?' He leaned over and kissed my cheek. 'You have some tools?'

My mind raced, trying to locate where I might have kept them, something so mechanical and functional like that so easy to forget. 'In the boot, I think. But honestly, you don't need to do this.'

'If I fix it, then you have a choice how you travel.'

My face flushed. I wasn't used to being on the receiving end of such kindness. I didn't know how to respond.

Outside, the air was freezing. Halloween lanterns flickered inside shop windows. Nikolaus had his head tucked under the car bonnet. We'd been standing in the car park for forty minutes, my cheeks ice cold, my hands warmed by the hot flask I held. I heard traffic in the distance.

After a while, feeling the cold moving into my body, I poured myself and Nikolaus a cup of tea. He popped his head out from under the car and slammed the bonnet shut.

'I think it is not so easy to fix it here,' he said, wiping his hands on an oil-smeared cloth. He grabbed the teacup. 'Can you drive to my place? I live on top of a garage. The owner is not there. I can fix it as you wait in the waiting area.'

He was concentrating, deadly focused on the job in hand. He was determined to get it done, no matter what. That glow and spark of his purpose, intent on helping me with whatever he could offer, made him even more attractive to me.

'Honestly, Nikolaus, I don't want to bother you. I'm embarrassed you're doing this.'

He laughed. 'Embarrassed, why? I told you: I want to.' He moved towards me and kissed me once more.

Seated in my car, we secured our seat belts. I placed the flask in a cup holder and rubbed my hands. 'Where exactly is this garage?' I asked. 'There's a risk the car won't make it.'

'From here, left, left, straight and right.'

I blinked.

'I show you.' He laughed. 'It is easier.'

Smiling, I turned on the ignition, pulling out of the car park. I drove cautiously onto the main road, thinking how nice it was to have Nikolaus sitting there beside me, his presence comforting and warm.

'Your radio is working?' he asked. We stopped at the lights, heading towards Civic Street.

'Sort of. It crackles. I don't use it much.' I turned left. Unusually, the roads were quiet, the car steady. I peered out into the darkness. Streaming shopfronts passed by, children holding their trick-or-treat buckets. 'It's Halloween tonight. And then, we move into Christmas.'

He nodded.

Was it too early for us to make plans concerning a date in the future?

'What will you do for Christmas?' I asked, determined to silence the downbeat voices in my head. Nikolaus was here, I so wanted to enjoy him.

He shrugged. 'I'm unsure. Sometimes I go to Heidelberg. Maybe this year I do something different.' He glanced at me, then turned, staring out of the window.

'We could . . . spend it together?'

From the corner of my eye, I saw him smile.

I bit my lip, thinking how different it would be to wake up on Christmas morning knowing there'd be someone special to spend it with.

'Sounds good,' he said.

We laughed as we turned right into Civic Street. 'Here,' he said, pointing to the corner.

I peered at the shops, taken aback when I saw the sign for Screaming Motors. I pressed the brake pedal, my foot suspended. 'You live in *there*?'

He nodded. 'I have a room at the top. You do not like it?'

'That's where Balraj was stabbed.'

'Yes. But I was not there.' He sighed. 'I heard about it, after. It was very terrible.' Nikolaus told me to pull into the back. Here, cars lined up for a service in an orderly and mechanical fashion.

'Why didn't you tell me your flat was on top of Screaming Motors?'

'I'm sorry. I did not think.' He turned to me. 'Of course, I see how the connection is important.'

I shook my head. 'Don't worry. I see how it was natural to overlook it.'

He clenched his jaw as if still berating himself.

'I open the back door and you can drive inside the garage,' he said, desperate to move on.

My mind scrambled to process the serendipitous nature of it all. All this time he lived here, and I didn't even know.

Nikolaus rolled up the shutter of the shop and I drove inside, still mulling things over. When he waved, I parked up, lifting the stiff handbrake.

I emerged from the car with a little hesitation. He was not lying when he said the place smelled of oil and petrol.

I threw Nikolaus my keys.

It was grey and cramped inside the garage, with room only for half a dozen vehicles. On either side, metal shelves were stocked with tins, sprays, plastic gallon containers. Nikolaus pointed to a worn velvet sofa in the corner. He moved to the side to switch on the heating; a fan whistled and whirred overhead. Soon, I felt the warm air relax me.

'I be quick. No one will know we are here,' he said.

I sat down, watching Nikolaus get to work. He rolled onto his back, carrying out an underbody inspection, scrambling to his feet after a few minutes to lift the car bonnet. He clanged his tools against the metal parts of the engine.

I pulled out my phone. Mercedes had sent me a text:

*Nina! I'm at a party. What are you doing? Want to come?*

I hesitated, not wanting to tell her I was with Nikolaus. It was too early. I wanted to keep this secret to myself.

I fired a message back.

*Bit tired, so having a quiet night.*

With the heat from the fan and the smell of fumes, I began to feel drowsy. I placed my phone down, resting my head against the armrest. I listened to the clinks and chinks of the screwdriver, to Nikolaus hammering his rubber mallet. I must have drifted off, waking only when my phone vibrated.

I swiped to answer the call.

'Nina! How are you doing sweeethaart?'

'Mercedes?' Most definitely it was her. She sounded drunk.

'Who else would it beee?'

'Have you been drinking?' I said.

'Whaaat? No! Why are yoo hasking?'

I laughed. 'Glad you're having fun. Who's with you – Sugar?'

I looked up and saw Nikolaus nod and smile. He ducked once again to continue working.

'I'm wiv Sssunil and . . . Rehggie, would you believe. Those boooys are proper mental. GOD heeelp me!'

I sat up, my ears ringing. 'You are? Can I speak to them – I need to talk to them about, you know, what we talked about, before.'

I felt my heart beating hard.

'Yepp! Hang on. I'll chat to Reg. I can go get Suuunil.' I heard a few muffled sounds, the loud RnB music in the background. 'Did you know, right, my maaate Neeena doesn't celebrate Halloweeeeen. She thinks it's too Americahnnn . . .'

'Mercedes!'

The line went dead.

I stood up, slipping the phone into my pocket, my breathing fast and shallow.

Nikolaus was standing before me, staring.

'Everything is okay?'

'Sure. That was just my friend, Mercedes.'

He nodded and ducked under the bonnet once more as I sent Mercedes a text.

*Tell Sunil I need to see him. Give him my number!!*

Within a minute, Sunil had sent me a text.

*What's up, Nina?*

I messaged him back.

*Can we meet? Got something serious I need to ask you. Tell me where and when. It won't take more than 30 mins!*

After around ten minutes I received a thumbs-up emoji and saw typing . . .

*Come round mine after the party if you want. Can't say I'll be in the best state for a conversation though!*

He texted me an address on the other side of town.

Nikolaus slammed down the bonnet and moved closer. 'It's done. Everything is fixed.' He wiped his hands on a paper towel, smiling.

Through my sleepy haze, I heard the car engine purr.

'What time is it?'

'Almost 2 a.m.,' he said.

'Really? That took *ages*. I am ever so grateful.'

Nikolaus looked pleased with himself. 'You had many problems, but I have resolved it.'

I ran into his arms and held him, kissing him several times on the cheek. 'You are such a kind man, Nikolaus. I don't know what I've done to deserve you.'

He laughed as I slipped into the driver's seat. I left the door open and Nikolaus stood outside, waiting for my reaction. But all I kept thinking about was Sunil. How I'd need to convince him to grant me access to Richard's emails – or to confidential files on his server. I needed to find something that linked Richard to MediCentral to expose his vested interest. I'd need to get numbers on how many tests had been carried out versus patients admitted. That would mean I'd need to access servers in phlebotomy . . .

My eyes blurred, mind raced. Inside my car, I gave Nikolaus the overreaction of an excited child. My hands trembled as they gripped the steering wheel. I placed my foot on the accelerator.

'She sounds good!' I called out of the open window.

I switched the engine off.

Nikolaus smiled. 'You want to go upstairs and sleep? I have spare clothes if you want a shower. But only if you want to . . .'

I bit my lip, tempted to say yes. But I shook my head because I knew I had to get home to see Sunil.

'It's late. I should get back,' I said.

Nikolaus's face fell.

'Why don't you come round tomorrow?' I said quickly.

'I check my rota,' he said, smiling.

Nikolaus waved as I pulled out of the garage into the car park. I drove onto the quiet street and heard the shutters close. I didn't look back. I was already thinking about Sunil and our meeting.

# 20

'What's this about? I've had a bit to drink. I've got a shift in the morning and need some sleep.'

The room around me was messy and stinking of weed. Sunil nodded at the faded velvet sofa and I sat down, careful to check there wasn't any dirt on the cushion. Just being in that front room, grey and smoky, made me feel light-headed.

'I need help. You're the only one I can speak to,' I said.

I stared around me, at how Sunil lived. His flat was shabby with two bedrooms. I heard movement in the second room, his flatmate, presumably. I tried not to judge, because, truth be told, I was no better.

Sunil grabbed a can of beer from the side. 'Want one?'

I shook my head. 'I'm driving.'

He pulled at the ring and the beer can opened with a fizz. He took a large gulp then sat down opposite me. 'Just want to say, I'm sorry to hear what happened.'

He stared down at the carpet, lost in thought. Just being with him, in his flat, seeing his face, hollow and worn out, reminded me of Newgate.

'There's stuff going on at Newgate. I'm looking into it. I feel like I'm caught up in a mess and if I don't do some digging, I'll be finished.' I stared down at my hands. They suddenly appeared old. 'There's a journalist involved. She will write about Newgate regardless. I need to give her the correct information. It's to help us all, or she'll trash us in the papers.'

'Why do you care, after what happened?'

'Because it's us she'll trash. Not the management. And I just know there's something going on.'

'Like *what*, exactly?'

'Like weird stuff going on since Richard's arrival – the way he's forced through changes and processes that affected us all . . . it stinks. How can anyone work for the good of patients with all that pressure? All his talk on generating revenue is bullshit.'

Sunil wiped his mouth on the corner of his sleeve. 'I've heard whispers. But we've just been told not to talk to journalists.'

'I've been suspended. So, therefore, I'm not listening.' I stood up, moving to the window, which was open. I closed my eyes, taking in the cold air. I inhaled deep, feeling it cold in my chest. 'I'm sorry to have to ask you this.' The early hours of the morning felt quiet and golden.

I saw Sunil ticking things over. 'And yet here you are.'

I nodded.

'Presumably what you're asking is IT-related?' he said.

'Richard's desktop access. And . . . phlebotomy.'

'You serious? CEO Richard. And phlebotomy?'

I pursed my lips. 'It's best I don't tell you too much.'

He snorted, then shrugged his shoulders. 'You need to be fucking careful, Nina.'

My stomach fluttered with excitement, knowing this was it, he was on board. 'So, you'll definitely help?'

'Depends.'

He glanced to the side, staring at a poster of a bhangra band on the wall.

'I'm being blamed for failures in care – and a patient died when I had nothing at all to do with it. It's important,' I said.

'I did hear. That's rough. Sorry, Nina. You don't deserve that.'

I glanced out onto the empty road lit up by the glow of a street lamp. A shop opposite was open. I watched the shopkeeper at the till, leaning on the counter, reading the paper.

'I still don't see the connection, though. Between you and . . . what the management are doing.' He took another sip of beer.

'Dev had so many tests before he died using a supplier that Richard brought in. But none of them were positive. How can that be? No one is questioning it.'

'So, you're saying they framed you. Made it look like you were negligent? What I heard is that you were distracted. That might just be rumours.'

I felt my insides clench. The thought of everyone talking about me made me feel sick. That sight of Leroy, whining in his bed, returned to me.

'People will always talk,' I said.

Sunil closed his eyes, leaning back into his chair. Eventually, he let out a long breath. 'I can't have this coming back to me.' He leaned forward. 'I mean it. It's dangerous. Criminal, even.'

'I swear – it won't.'

'I'm getting out. So, I'll see what I can do. Don't give a fuck what happens, to tell the truth.'

I wanted to hug him. 'Where will you go?'

'Maybe move into retail management. Pays better.'

I nodded, overcome with sadness that it had come to this. Good, solid workers like Sunil broken and fed up working in the NHS.

I stood up, ready to leave, feeling like I'd already asked too much of him. 'I'm so grateful,' I said.

He grunted. 'We'll organise a time and I'll log you on. The beauty about IT is that it can all be remote. You need to be quick, though, yeah? I'll give you limited time. Fifteen minutes, maximum.'

I nodded, taking that as my cue to move to the door. 'What if I need more time?'

'You could go into his office, use his fixed workstation. There, I'd give you around thirty minutes.'

I opened the front door. 'I don't know how to thank you.'

He shuffled behind me, hands wedged firmly in his pockets. 'There is one thing you could do,' he said.

I turned, staring into his face, waiting for what might be an unreasonable request. There must be a catch. There's always a catch. 'What is it?'

'Your mate Mercedes . . .'

'What about her?'

'Could you put in a good word?'

The next day, having slept soundly with the comfort of a working car, knowing that my plans to collect evidence were finally paying off, I walked a few yards down Old-field Lane. I heard devotional songs of holy hymns, kirtan delivered by tablas, beaten by a heavy palm. Breathy har-monium notes, enlivened by the power of men's voices. I didn't understand a word, but the music was raw, alive with emotion.

I'd run out of food again. At the Guru Nanak Gurdwara, they offered a free meal to help carry me through. The sign on the door to the yellow building read *Everyone is Welcome.*

From inside the lobby, with its navy carpet, brilliant-white walls chequered with paintings of golden temples and Gurumukhi scrawls, I made my way into the Langar Hall.

*Balraj.*

This was where he prayed, his heart pouring with devotion, gratitude, and appreciation of life's complications. I felt my heart sink into my stomach knowing he'd been viciously attacked. Resentment rose, like gushing water on the street from a burst water pipe. That sight of Leroy, his barbed-wire tattoo. The audacity of his entitlement, prioritisation, at the expense of other good, hard-working people.

My phone vibrated. Nikolaus had sent me a text:

*Hope the car was okay last night. I am missing you already. Thank you for the delicious pasta. x*

I collected a silver tray from the side and waited in line for a meal. There were three curries to choose from: cauliflower, spinach, and chickpeas. Rice and roti was offered as an accompaniment. A row of five men with long grey beards, silky turbans, spooned piles of food onto my plate. The man at the end with gold-rimmed glasses asked whether I wanted Indian tea or just water with it.

'Tea, please.'

Balancing my tray in my hands, I moved to the back of the hall. Everyone sat cross-legged on a single white sheet laid flat on the floor. I shuffled closer so I wouldn't have to eat alone, feeling an overwhelming sense of comfort just then, dwelling anonymously among locals. Everyone here was like me, struggling to get through the day, to make ends meet.

A cold draught entered the hall as the doors swung open. A breeze wafted; Community Kitchen posters ruffled.

Two uniformed police officers shuffled into the queue. One of them, I recognised as the novel-reading officer watching over Leroy at Newgate.

To my left, a man in a velvet suit was watching me eat. His eyes narrowed as if trying to place me.

I struggled to chew my food, knowing he was there. My stomach clenched when I saw him approaching.

'You are from the hospital, yes?' He stared down at me, his face fatherly and warm. I caught a whiff of his jacket, cinnamon mingled with cardamon.

'I'm a nurse,' I said. But as I said those words, they hurt. 'I work at Newgate.' Except, of course, I wasn't there now . . .

He smiled knowingly, sympathetically, meeting my eyes with his, strawberry pink, milky with cataracts. I wondered whether I'd seen him around too, unable to establish whether he'd been a patient, or perhaps a visitor.

'My mother was in the hospital last month,' he said, 'you people were very kind. But she died because of the long waiting times.'

I dropped my spoon.

'It is not your fault. We know how it is. We were angry, but now we have accepted it.'

I nodded, tearing a piece of roti, folding it with my fingers. What was he going to say? That he knew about Dev? That I was indeed useless and negligent?

'In my mother's name, I would like to give you something.' He fumbled around in his pocket and held out a twenty-pound note. 'For you, take it.'

I was taken aback. 'I can't possibly take that,' I said. 'You don't know half of it, I feel really bad.' I placed my roti on my plate. 'Not after what happened . . . what I did. It wouldn't be right.'

He looked at me, perplexed. 'But my mother would want you to have it, to say thank you. You are not to blame. It is the government. They do not organise things properly. I don't know . . . maybe now, with a new prime minister, things will be different.' He tutted, pressing the note into my palm. 'Please.'

I felt the note crisp in my hand. My fingers clenched as my eyes watered. 'I'm sorry . . . about your mother . . . and for every other patient suffering . . .'

'She was old. Ninety-four. When old people die, it is easier to accept. She had a good life, and she lived it.' He smiled.

My stomach warmed as he disappeared.

Inside my flat, my stomach full, I took a seat at the kitchen table and pulled out my phone. Still nothing from Sunil. But I knew he wouldn't let me down. I scrolled through my emails and saw I'd received a new message from Barbara:

*Appreciate this is a difficult time and that everyone is under enormous strain, but we'd like to discuss the outcome of the investigation into Dev Shah's death. It's important we do this in person. Would you be able to attend a meeting with myself and the management team? This has been scheduled for Wednesday 2nd November 2022 at 3 p.m. Maria will be sharing her findings. Do feel free to bring a representative.*

The tone of it was warm at least, compassionate with even a hint of understanding. That was something, coming from Barbara, whose twenty years as a healthcare professional had, no doubt, turned her wooden. All I kept thinking was, *this is it*. They must have found something worse – maybe realised I'd stolen morphine. Most likely they'd blame me for Dev's death. Or maybe it was nothing. Maybe I'd be cleared.

I sent Sunil a text to hurry him along:

*Any news when? It's getting a bit urgent.*

After a minute, he replied:

*I can give you 15 minutes in around 2 hours. I've checked and it's all clear.*

My heart began beating faster as I glanced around for my tablet. I replied:

*What do I do exactly?*

Three dots appeared . . . and then a reply:

*On an Android device, download the Chrome Remote Desktop app. Will send you a link. Do this by 3 p.m. NO LATER. Will then send you instructions and a pin just before. You've got 15 mins only, from exactly 3 p.m. today – Ok??*

I swallowed hard. Within seconds, he'd sent me a link.

I grabbed my tablet from the sofa and began downloading the app. My connection was a bit slow, so I used my phone to distract myself.

I clicked onto www.levinstonematters.com to read the latest comments:

Sukh_52:
*What is happening to our kids these days??? What is their and our future!? We emigrated to UK in the early 70s and sure, it was hard for us, so we developed a community to support each other and to protect ourselves from racism. But we had boundaries – and a code. For these gangs, it's all about drugs and violence, using minors to do their selling. Where the hell are the police? I'm seriously considering whether we move on. The UK dream is broken!*

CynthiaPerris:
*I read somewhere the Met are now arresting people using live facial recognition technology . . . shop owners are installing it. Brilliant, I say. Lock 'em up. But we still need the police to do their jobs. The tech does not work on gangs wearing masks or balaclavas*

*or when groups jump on innocent people!*

Matt90:
*I am very worried about my children going to school. So many of them are vaping. Where are they getting it from??*

SandraZ:
*Facial recognition is NOT the answer!! It can make errors and wrongly match your face with someone who might have committed a crime. Next thing you know, the police are knocking on your door, arresting you for a crime you didn't commit. The reality is that it will be mainly black men arrested!*

RightSaidFred99:
*These kids need a place to let off steam. Or they will get themselves injured or killed then clog up our 'free' services!! And guess who will have to cough up the bill? UK TAXPAYERS!*

About to log off, I noticed a 'like' under a post for a new shopping centre opening in Lyndon Hill – R Lonsdale.

I opened Google, typed in his name and scrolled through listings before locating Richard Lonsdale's Facebook profile. The page was unloved, mostly abandoned. The last post was in 2016: a wedding photo of a woman in a lace-trimmed wedding dress, linking arms with a rotund, smiley-faced man in a wedding suit. *My beautiful little sister's wedding*, read the caption.

The names of the couple tagged were Sophie Lonsdale and Mark Dickson. I clicked on Mark Dickson's page. He was a director, it said. Medical research. Was that the personal connection that Mary had told Mercedes about in relation to MediCentral?

My phone vibrated. Another text came in from Sunil:

*Done?*

I checked my tablet. By now it was two thirty. The app was sixty-five per cent downloaded. I typed a return message:

*Almost. Will be done by 3 p.m., I think. 35% left.*

On my phone, I searched for MediCentral online. Their website appeared clinical and cold. The landing page revealed the company dealt in medical devices and remote testing solutions. On the 'About' page, I saw information on 'Purpose and Values', 'Corporate Responsibility', 'Environmental', 'Social and Governance'. After a few seconds, I spotted a small tab that said 'Board'.

I clicked onto the Board page, saw their CEO at the top. A bald man with spectacles, plus their CFO, MD. But not Mark Dickson.

I sighed. But continued searching.

I looked up MediCentral on Companies House. The registered office address was in Farnham. Incorporated on 22nd July 2015. Under People, I searched for their list of directors, and that's when it finally appeared.

Three directors listed – one of them none other than Mark Dickson.

I slammed my phone down; I couldn't believe it. Mark was Richard's brother-in-law, married to his sister, Sophie, and in charge of MediCentral. Richard, Newgate's CEO, had forced MediCentral's appointment and introduced off-site testing – because there was a family connection. A connection he was most likely benefiting from. For a split second, I panicked. I wondered whether Mercedes was right about all this being dangerous.

It was 2.55 p.m. Sunil sent me another text with a PIN and a set of instructions.

My hands trembled as my fingers swept over the tablet.

I logged in and watched as Richard's desktop appeared on my screen. On the left, a yellow shortcut folder to the hospital drive. Double-clicking, I scanned down the letters:

Local Disk (C:)
Archive (Q:)
Administration (B:)
Finance (F:)
Management (M:)

There were too many folders. I clicked on Management.

I wanted to see if there was any correspondence connecting Richard to anyone there, to prove a conflict of interest. But searching through the folders, I found nothing.

I went to his email inbox. Typed in 'blood testing, MediCentral, Mark Dickson, supplier engagement'.

The first thing I saw was an email Richard had received from HR. Subject: Confidential Restructures.

September 1, 2022

*Richard, further to our chat, I've now developed a phased plan. Would be good to discuss in person. I'll put in some time.*
*Matthew Wright*
*Chief of Staff*

I was trawling now as fast as I could, desperate for anything – anything relating to MediCentral. My heart skipped a beat when I finally saw an email marked 'Private'. It was from M Dickson and simply read:

June 1, 2022

*R, Glad we could make this work. See you at ours at the weekend.*
*Mark*

I swallowed. *Could this be it?* The email was via Gmail – and was also cc'd to Richard's personal Gmail account: RL76@gmail.com.

It was all I could find. It simply wasn't enough. I needed proof that he'd given MediCentral preferential treatment by awarding the contract, although the connection to Mark alone was damning.

By now it was 3.14 p.m. and I had no choice but to log off. I forwarded the email to my personal account and went to Richard's sent folder to delete evidence of my doing it.

I sent Sunil a text:

*I'm going to need ACTUAL access.*

He sent a reply:

*Ok I'll try – but this is the last thing I'm doing.*

I logged out of my tablet and placed it on the table, face down. Closing my eyes, I tried to settle my racing heart. It was unbelievable. Richard Lonsdale had a nerve. There were consequences for others he'd not even bothered to think about.

I showered and dressed, gulping down a mug of tea alongside two ibuprofen tablets. I had a stonking headache and needed sleep. But as I tried to put my head down, I felt restless, unable to stop tossing and turning. My sleep patterns were a mess. Having trained myself to sleep during the day, my body now resisted it.

All I could think about was the audacity and downright entitlement of Richard, to assume he could hire his own, while evading detection. There *must* be something more that proved he financially profited from the deal. I simply had to find it.

Around eight thirty there was a knock on the door.

'Put the kettle on, I'd love to catch up.' Mercedes barged in, throwing down her coat, but she stopped suddenly, after taking only a few steps forward.

'What the hell is going on in here? This place is a tip!'

I glanced around me as Mercedes moved nearer, placing the back of her hand to my forehead. 'You must be sick. Temperature seems fine, and yet, there's no way the Nina *I* know would live like this.'

She was right. I had let everything go. The overwhelm of the last few days – and certainly the events earlier – had fettered me, leaving me clinging on to a metal pole. My discovery about Richard burned deep into my core. I had bigger things to focus on now.

'I was going to tidy up,' I said. 'But I've been called in.'

'When?'

'Wednesday at 3 p.m.'

'What for? Did they say?'

'The outcome of the investigation.' Saying it out loud brought home its importance.

'Don't worry. I'll come to you straight afterwards. I'll meet you on the ward, if you like.'

There was a pile of dirty clothes overflowing the laundry basket. The sink was full of dirty dishes. Flyers, leaflets, newspapers lay scattered over the unvacuumed carpet. I got up and stared down at it all.

*Disgusting.*

Mercedes sighed. She stood behind me and threw her car keys onto the side table. 'Look, I don't have much time. I just wanted to make sure you were okay. Did you speak to Sunil?'

'I did. He said he'll help. I'm waiting for details.'

I got up to turn the kettle on, my head throbbing. I couldn't get into it now. Mercedes would be dramatic, and besides, it was too dangerous for her to know too much. I needed harder evidence. I needed time to think.

'Nina, are you sure about this?'

'I know what I'm doing,' I mumbled.

'But the meeting. At least wait to hear what they say.'

*The meeting*. She was right. Deep down, I knew it might not end well.

I tried to keep positive, thinking of Nikolaus, how he'd fixed my car. How lovely that felt.

The kettle boiled. I made us both tea.

I handed Mercedes a mug and she cupped it with both hands.

'What can I do to help?' she asked. 'I feel a bit useless.'

I sat down, crossing my legs, sipping from my mug. 'It's better you stay out of it. I don't want you getting into trouble as well.'

Mercedes' mouth downturned.

'Okay, fine. I looked Richard Lonsdale up online. Turns out he has a brother-in-law in medical research – can you believe?'

'You serious?'

I grabbed my phone and opened Facebook, handing it over to Mercedes, watching her face pale.

She shook her head, tutting. 'Doesn't prove anything specific, though, does it?'

I clenched my jaw. 'There's a family connection. He *must* be benefiting from it. Why would he have forced Medi-Central in, otherwise?'

'I'm not sure . . . I just don't know how you go about proving something like that.' She went on to admire Sophie's wedding dress, said she liked the trim. She was about to return my phone when it vibrated.

'It's Sunil,' Mercedes said nervously.

I grabbed it, staring down at the message.

*Midnight. Tomorrow. Reggie will sort it.*

# 21

Outside Heartbeat, I waited for Maria to let me in. She opened the meeting-room door coyly, lowering her eyes as I entered.

Inside, the moody sky was visible through the large, sparkling windows. It appeared so beautiful and serene, this view of the town from the top, minus the street-level details.

I positioned myself at the centre of the conference table, aware of the prickling unease in the air. It was surprising how many of them were in attendance. *One functional team*, like organs connected to pronounce judgement.

'I appreciate this must be difficult,' said Barbara. 'Thanks for coming in at such short notice.'

I tried to make myself comfortable, but my stomach was in knots.

Directly opposite sat Peter Jones, Newgate's new head of nursing – narrow face, dry, orange-peel skin. We'd hardly spoken. The fact that he was here spoke volumes about how serious this all was. His eyes that said he'd seen this all before, women supposedly like me, who start out wide-eyed in nursing, optimistic, motivated to give something back, before slowly growing disillusioned.

A good nurse turned bad, perhaps.

I clutched either side of my seat then leaned forward to assert my presence more powerfully. 'I want to make it clear that I don't feel I've done anything wrong,' I said.

They looked at one another.

Peter cleared his throat. 'Well, good to know where you stand. It's important you hear the conclusion of our findings, and the implications for you, personally. I appreciate this might be a little overwhelming.' Peter shuffled in his seat. 'Having us all here, like this. But do take it as a compliment that we're taking *this*, and *you*, seriously.' He smiled, though somehow, only his lips moved.

Barbara twirled the ends of her curls between her fingers.

'We'll keep it brief, to allow us more time for a conversation.' That was Matthew Wright, chief of staff. Grey suit. Dotted tie. Slapped in the face with the wet fish of a divorce he claimed he didn't deserve because it was all down to his ex-wife. 'Of course, you'll have an opportunity to respond, before we conclude with an outcome.'

I nodded, suddenly overcome with a sense of foreboding. Everything felt so final and incriminating.

'Maria, would you begin?' Matthew leaned back in his seat. Maria smiled and I thought I saw something, a flash – a look, of quiet satisfaction – sweeping across her face.

She peered down at her notes. 'Of course. We're here to outline the findings of the seventy-two-hour mandatory investigation into Mr Dev Shah's death on 25th October, 1 a.m., and further to the discrepancies we've already mentioned to you, Nina, during your shift on Thursday 27th October. Is there anything you'd like to ask me, or to clarify, before we begin?'

I shook my head.

'I'll take that as *no*.' Maria sounded like a barrister in front of a jury.

'Mr Dev Shah arrived in A&E on Thursday 20th October at 8 a.m. with severe stomach pains. He was triaged with essential tests carried out. All returned negative, upon which it was confirmed he should receive an appendectomy – precautionary only – and be admitted to ASU while awaiting surgery. To confirm, he was admitted to ASU at approximately 10 p.m. on the 20th, while a space in theatre was made available.'

'The same day – after *fourteen* hours!' clarified Peter.

'Yes,' said Barbara.

'*Christ*.'

The adrenalin raced. I couldn't hold back. 'That waiting time is unacceptable, I know. But it's only one of the ways that lack of staff is failing our patients.'

Barbara held up her hand, motioning for me to stay quiet. 'We're aware,' she said, 'but that is a different point. Maria, please, let's continue.'

Maria turned a page.

'Dev was allocated to ASU because no spaces were available on the appropriate ward. Delays in admission into ASU and delays in theatre meant that Dev Shah did not receive an operation until 1 p.m. on Friday 21st October. He returned to ASU after four hours, at 5.06 p.m. He complained of stomach pains and was seen by Dr Milburn, on duty at the time. Dr Milburn prescribed him two doses of morphine, 10mg each.'

'I wasn't there for that.' I could not shut up. 'I started my shift at eight that evening. Also, I had a conversation with his mother, Manisha Shah, and she said he mustn't take those morphine tablets. He needed to be seen by a doctor.

She wanted him to be given a firm diagnosis before taking medication. That's also why Dev didn't take the other ones, which were misplaced.'

I knew I'd stolen those second tablets, but I didn't care. They were obviously stitching me up. What difference would it make?

Maria pursed her lips, ignoring me. I had an overwhelming urge to slap her.

'Dev Shah was seen by Dr Milburn at 10.04 p.m.,' she continued. 'A decision was taken to carry out a CT scan and to keep Dev under observation. Morphine was further prescribed, a course of eight tablets, 10mg each to be taken every six hours as needed. A record of it is missing in his medication chart, which is strange. Dr Milburn is sure he wrote it down.'

'I see,' said Peter.

'Nina mentioned, after Dev's death, that she'd applied hydrocortisone cream to a rash Dev developed that night. She also administered a Piriton tablet. That seems to have been omitted, also.' Maria added that with a hint of sarcasm.

'On the 22nd, Nina worked her shift in the evening. Dev received an FBC at 9 a.m. and a CT scan later that morning, which appeared normal. Nina carried out a further FBC at 9 p.m. On 23rd October, it appears that Nina was off. Dev Shah was seen by Sandra Willis and a nurse from Platinum Care. A repeat of those tests took place to see if there were any changes. On the 24th, Nina returned to work for her shift and carried out the usual obs.'

'Why were so many tests necessary? Maybe we should talk about that!'

‘All tests returned negative,’ clipped Maria. ‘Worth noting that, having carried out a post-mortem, there is no evidence of morphine in Dev’s bloodstream. No tablets found, either. Most likely they were removed from the premises, although of course we can’t prove it.’

‘Surely the issue is that Dev died, that nothing showed up in *any* of the tests to help us understand why – despite him having so many of them. The morphine is a minor issue!’ I added.

Maria glared at me. ‘It’s all relevant, at this point,’ she said. ‘Even those minor points, because a *death* is involved.’

‘Hang on, let’s slow it down. Do we have the sequence of events for the 23rd when Nina was off?’ asked Peter.

Maria shuffled through her notes. ‘We do, yes. Sandra Willis was interviewed. Nothing unusual found in the obs. Dev Shah was Nina’s patient. She was simply covering for her.’

‘And was Dev seen by a doctor?’ I pressed.

Barbara said, ‘Yes. At noon. All clear. Nothing of concern. It was Dr Milburn.’

Maria paused and consulted her notes. ‘In terms of the sequence of events on Tuesday 25th October 2022, Mr Dev Shah died at 1 a.m. The coroner’s report suggests cause of death to be SCD – sudden cardiac death – during Dev’s sleep. This is *not* considered to be suspicious. This leads me to confirm that no further medical investigation is required concerning Dev’s death.’

I released a long exhale and leaned back in my chair. ‘Thank God,’ I said. ‘I’m so relieved. You can’t imagine how worried I’ve been. But we still need to understand why it happened. He was so young.’

But no one else shared my concern.

Maria cleared her throat. 'An investigation *is* required concerning the care Dev received during his inpatient stay, under Nina's supervision.'

The room fell silent. I suddenly felt sick.

'We've identified failures when carrying out duties. The issue of morphine missing is also extremely serious. Action was taken when our initial suspicions arose, when Nina was suspended on full pay on Thursday 27th October, to allow us more time to investigate.'

Barbara turned. 'Is there anything you'd like to say, at this point?' I saw her eyes had turned cold, reptilian.

I shook my head, unable to think of anything to say.

'Do continue,' Peter said.

'There are four areas of concern,' said Maria, 'which Dev's untimely death has highlighted.'

'You do understand, don't you?' asked Matthew, turning to me, 'how serious this is?'

I nodded, determined not to lose it. I needed to let them talk, though I knew where all this was heading. I saw a flash of Dev in the mortuary, his skin mottled with smears of blue on his face. It didn't make sense – then or now. There had to be more to it.

Matthew cleared his throat and folded his arms. 'You've declined to have a representative present, which, of course, is your choice entirely . . .'

Until that point, I hadn't felt the need to have anyone with me to fight my corner.

Maria straightened her back.

'The first issue – the biggest issue – is the morphine discrepancy, which we've already mentioned.' Maria glanced at me. 'Morphine was prescribed but there's no record of it – and it was not administered. This is particularly suspicious because it has transpired that there are morphine discrepancies in Florence Nightingale, namely an increase in sign-outs in the ledger by persons not known. On days when Nina was on duty. Not huge amounts, but enough to raise suspicion. Those suspicions were reported to Nina by Ravi Patel, the ward's pharmacist, but were *not* relayed to Matron Barbara Dean, despite a request to do so, and despite Nina's assurance that she would pass on the information.'

I bit my tongue.

'There are also other areas of concern, regarding conduct.' Maria looked down. 'Just before arriving in ASU, the operations manager, Jimmi Rangoon, enquired whether there were any vacant beds for Dev Shah. Two were available at the time, but Nina said there were none.'

I picked at a scab on my hands and drew blood. 'It was a simple mistake,' I spat. 'An administrative error.'

'Did you confirm it was an error to Jimmi?' asked Barbara, her voice harder.

I nodded, gloating. 'I did.'

'There's more,' said Maria.

*Of course there was more. That stupid bitch.*

'We've had reports of concerning views expressed in regard to the admission of patients.'

'What does that mean?' I asked, dumbfounded.

'Yes, what *does* that mean?' asked Peter.

'Views concerning which patients should and should not receive treatment.'

'Good grief,' Peter said.

'Views which are in breach of fundamental nursing ethics, and which undermine the spirit of our National Health Service.'

Peter glanced down, shaking his head.

*They're talking about Leroy. Sandra has said something.*

'In speaking to staff on the ward, some have stated they've witnessed from Nina . . . how should I put it . . . *antagonistic behaviour* towards patients. Belittling them, teasing them, threatening them, even.'

It was the final blow. I knew then it was game over. No matter what was going on, I didn't stand a chance. Look how many of them there were. I also remembered what Barbara said on the night of my suspension, that they wouldn't get the NMC involved. That had to be because they couldn't prove any of the accusations made.

'This is so unfair. You called me into a meeting to confirm Dev's death – which I had nothing to do with. But now you're accusing me of failings in my duty of care. I know that, maybe, I could have been more professional. That it was unacceptable not to have notes accurate. But I never hurt Dev. I'm not responsible for his death. You need to focus on what's really going on.'

Barbara glanced awkwardly at the others.

'All I wanted was to do my job,' I said, my eyes stinging. 'But this hospital has made it impossible because of the way it operates.'

My hands wouldn't stop twitching in my lap. I gulped mouthfuls of air, trying to keep it all in. I told myself to breathe . . . to breathe slow and steady, to not say anything until I had enough evidence.

'Regardless of your good intention, a line was crossed. With Leroy, for example. We cannot ignore it.' Barbara's brow arched. 'It was part of your training as a nurse. One of the very first things you covered. *Ethics. Selfless service. Indiscriminate care.*'

'And so, inevitably, there are consequences,' said Matthew.

The word *consequences* hung like a noose in the air.

I placed a hand over my face.

As they read over the terms of my severance, I was not sure if the words sank in. I heard the words *termination*, gross misconduct, dummy words that filled a page, but that carried no meaning.

'I'll speak to the RCN,' I said. 'I'll get legal advice. I'll protect myself!'

'Of course, you should do that,' said Barbara.

They turned their attention to their notes. It was an employment matter, they said. I'd need legal advice if I wanted to appeal. I was lucky the issues were not being reported to the NMC, nor a record of it logged on the register, which risked my professional licence. They made a point of reiterating that I was being let go with immediate effect, with only the remainder of this month's salary paid. This, given the circumstances, was generous.

Peter nodded and I stood up, my shirt crumpled like crêpe paper. Outside the meeting room, I gasped, as if all this time I'd been denied fresh air.

The others filed out. Peter and Matthew slipped into the next room. I caught a quick glimpse of Richard seated on a sofa as the door opened, like he might have been waiting for them.

Barbara escorted me back to the ward, and as I walked into the changing room, she waited outside. I texted Mercedes to meet me, then stuffed my bag with the remaining items from my locker: an old cardigan, a half-empty box of tampons, Cup a Soup, a pad of Post-it notes. I didn't look up when I saw Sandra enter. She stood behind me.

'I'm so sorry,' she said, 'really, I am. I know you've been through a lot.'

'Fuck off,' I replied. 'I know you've been talking about me behind my back.'

I watched her face fall, and then, as if convincing herself that I was simply troubled, she bent down to pick up a fallen hairband. She reached out, handing it to me.

'I never meant to cause any problems. I did what I had to. We need to put patients first, Nina. No matter how difficult.'

I laughed, snatching the hairband from her. 'I love how you're now so *senior*, so expert! Are you still a nurse, or suddenly qualified to be a doctor?'

At that precise moment, Mercedes barged in. 'Nina! Is everything okay?' She took one look at my face and knew what it meant.

She rushed into my arms, the warm, cocoa-butter scent of her providing comfort. Sandra shook her head and moved to the corner, shuffling out. Mercedes and I were alone, and we stared at one another as the door closed.

'Tonight,' said Mercedes turning to me. 'Are you still doing it?'

The tears trickled down my face, gasps rose from the deepest part of my chest. 'I am now *so* determined. You were right. This place isn't worth it.' My shoulders juddered. 'I gave them too much and look where it got me.'

'I feel terrible,' said Mercedes, taking a seat on the wooden bench. She placed her hand on my bag and fastened the top. 'I don't like where this is heading.'

I sat down next to her. 'What choice do I have?'

She thought for a moment. Then she asked, 'Did they confirm how Dev died?'

'SDC – but nothing suspicious. They're letting me go on gross misconduct but keeping it internal.'

Mercedes shook her head. 'Want to meet up later and talk about it?'

But I no longer wanted to talk. I searched around the changing room to make sure I hadn't left anything behind. Mercedes nodded and left me to it as I picked up my bag.

I rushed out, leaving Barbara trailing behind me.

Outside, I lumbered down the steps, the air oppressive, striking my cheeks. I carried on walking without looking back.

# 22

Richard Lonsdale's office was on the top floor. The airless corridor was long and dark. Golden light from the street lamps outside splintered across the carpet.

Carefully, I selected the skeleton key that Reggie had marked for me with a red sticker from the bunch he'd handed over during our brief meeting. He'd said the other keys *might come in handy* once I was in. He didn't want to ask any questions about what I was doing.

I slid the key into the lock; it was stiff. I grabbed the handle and turned it. Initially, the door didn't move. I tried the key once more, this time with a softer twist, a little lift. I heard it click open.

The door swept over the thick carpet; the air inside was stuffy. The walls around me seemed to speak, promising to keep my deepest secrets.

I switched on the torch on my phone, holding it out, watching the silver light streak over the walls and ceiling. I crept towards the window with its open blinds and stood closer to the moonlight.

There were six wheelie chairs around a conference table, each tilted as if people had risen in a hurry from an urgent meeting. On the wall, a framed print of a tiger. A stack of files lay at the edge of the table, a few pencils scattered.

So, this is where it happened, I thought. The oily decision-making that kept the conveyor belt of the hospital factory moving. I held my breath, taking it all in, continuing to the far-right corner where Richard's desk was. I swept my hand over the warm, glassy surface. Glancing up, I took a deep breath, throwing light towards the door to make doubly sure I'd closed it.

I switched the torch off and turned his computer on. Within seconds, the screen blinked into life.

My hands trembled as my fingers swept over the keyboard. I logged in with the password Sunil had shared with me earlier: *RLons49781#&!*

Richard's desktop flashed up looking exactly as I'd seen it before. I had thirty minutes. I needed to be quick. But thirty minutes was not enough time to find something specific.

I scanned Richard's list of drives once more, but they revealed nothing new. I clicked onto a new drive, Local Disk (C:), figuring that maybe he'd hide something in there since it was accessible only to him.

Inside was a folder labelled 'Finance' with another folder inside it, labelled 'Suppliers'. It took a few minutes, but tucked in among Word and .xls files, I found a contract, which confirmed MediCentral's appointment in August 2022. Scanning the terms, I found it had a deadline for roll-out in October the same year. I opened and then closed it. This told me nothing I didn't know. I needed something explosive.

I was feeling the pressure of the clock ticking, and I began to search Richard's desk for anything that resembled official paperwork. There were medical journals, a pile of reports. I opened the drawers on either side and began rummaging through them. The left drawer was full of Post-its, six cereal bars, a shopping receipt for wine and beers from Waitrose. Two small bottles of Evian. But on my right, underneath a black conference folder containing an A4 pad and calculator, I found a small notebook. I opened it up, scanning the pages. There was a list. The entries appeared to be a log of passwords for online accounts. One entry read Santander.

My heart raced.

I went to the homepage in Richard's browser and attempted to log in, hoping that his details might be stored and, somehow, I might be able to enter. On Santander's home page, his Personal ID appeared, 0024873797. But it was clear I needed a security number to access his account. I glanced at the notebook and saw a line of numbers under '£'. I entered it and within seconds, I was able to log in.

I saw Richard's monthly salary: £20,833.33. I felt sick as I scanned the rest of the entries. He was a fan of coffee, that was for sure – spending £4.40 each day in Costa. A couple of big mortgages were there, too – one for £7,527.93 to Barclays, and another for £3,254.76 to Halifax. But it was the entries marked MediCentral that caught my eye. Each month, from MediCentral's contractual appointment in August 2022, to now, a credit appeared. In August, he'd received £15,000. In September, £15,550. In October, £20,987.00 – which was when the roll-out began.

That appearance of MediCentral on the statement was enough to confirm corruption. I felt my head pound as it sank in. This was it. Clear evidence of some sort of back-hander. Those differing amounts each month screamed that Richard was being incentivised – paid more, the more testing we did. No wonder he'd forced outsourcing bloods onto Newgate. He didn't give a damn about patients.

I'd got what I needed. I downloaded the statement and printed it off.

The printer groaned and clicked as it warmed up. My stomach clenched upon hearing the noise.

I had ten minutes left. In the notebook, I found the log-in details for a Gmail account. Next, I attempted to log in using the details logged: RL76@gmail.com, password, Richard Lon_1498@!

I saw the same email I'd read before, that one from Mark thanking Richard for 'making this work'. *See you at ours at the weekend.* Those words made my head rush.

I clicked on the sent box and found another email from Richard to Mark, dated just after that one.

June 2, 2022

*M,*
*Likewise. I'm assuming we can agree terms as discussed based on volumes? If all goes well, we'll extend.*
*RL*

*Unbelievable.*

I forwarded the emails to my own Hotmail account, careful to delete any trace I'd done it. I couldn't wait to tell Mercedes about this. Finally, I had hard evidence.

Twenty-five minutes had passed. I needed to get out.

I logged out, switching off the machine, rushed out of the

office and locked the door; I heard voices in the distance as I ran towards the fire exit and made my way down the stairs.

Outside, as the cold air entered my lungs, I steadied myself and grabbed my phone.

By now, it was 12.35 a.m. I dialled Farah's number, and she answered.

'Who is it?' I heard the sound of a ruffling blanket.

I paused as I rushed out of the car park onto the main road.

'It's Nina. I've got it!' I was breathless, running. 'I've got what you need for a story to prove corruption at Newgate!'

'Nina? Jesus! What time is it?'

'Evidence of a sure conflict of interest in the appointment of a supplier. MediCentral, brought in to handle routine and gold standard blood testing. I have an email to prove one of the directors is his brother-in-law. Richard has been getting kickbacks – personally profiting from MediCentral's appointment. Can you believe it? I have a bank statement to prove it.'

I heard her jump out of bed. 'Wait. Slow down! Bank statements – and emails? Are you sure? Oh my God.'

'Mark Dickson, a director at MediCentral, is married to Richard's sister, Sophie! See what you think. I'm almost home. I'll email you everything.'

'This is great, Nina. Really great.' I heard Farah breathing fast.

'But this can't get back to me, do you hear?' I said. 'You wanted a story – and I got you one. This is big, trust me.'

'I'm a woman of my word.'

'I mean it, Farah.'

'I promise!' she said, laughing almost.

I was rushing now, racing to my car, parked on a street corner outside a Turkish kebab shop.

'Also, just to make it clear, I have nothing to do with Dev's death. Do you hear me? The internal investigation states SCD. So don't go dragging my name in the mud. You want to be writing about this instead. It's criminal!'

Farah was silent.

'Are you listening?' I shouted.

I was inside my car, the phone pressed to my ear. I tucked it onto my shoulder as I thrust the key into the ignition.

'Got it,' she said, a little too late.

'I need to go,' I said. 'I very much look forward to reading what you write.'

Farah laughed at my smugness as I pulled out from the kerb.

'Don't you worry,' she said. 'Just send me what you have. I'll have a look and then discuss it, first thing, with my editor. If you have what you say you do, then *wow*.'

'I do,' I said.

'In that case, you've got nothing to worry about.'

# 23

Life is just a series of breaths. Inside my flat, my chest rising and falling, breaths quick and shallow, all I could do now was wait. I'd taken huge risks to gather the evidence I did, to email it to Farah. But now, I was left waiting for something to happen.

I'd never thought about the nature or movement of time when working in a hospital. Hours packed with urgent examinations, diagnoses, treatments. But now, cooped up in my flat, jobless, time moved slowly. It was like wading through congealed mud in a rain-sodden field.

In that space, sinking deeper into the emptiness, the silence, thoughts began to overwhelm me. They pulled me into a dark and destructive corner where Leroy was seated, taunting me, reminding me that, despite Balraj lying paralysed, he'd gotten away with it. Just thinking of Leroy in that hospital bed, his snarly grin, his prioritisation and downright *entitlement*, got me fired up. Despite all the issues at Newgate, I would have managed to overcome them had he not been there distracting me. Now I'd lost my job. No longer was I a nurse – because of him. Dev might still be alive. In the depths of my despair, stripped of my identity, a new and dangerous narrative formed . . .

However illogical it might seem, Leroy became a symbol of everything I despised. Everything gone wrong. The one half of my identity I'd denied and hated, embodied in this one man.

I moved to the window, the afternoon air grey and cloudy. I desperately needed to eat. I grabbed my bag, only to discover that inside was a pink Post-it attached to a fifty-pound note. I recognised that spidery handwriting as belonging to Mercedes:

*Get yourself a treat. Don't think any more about them!*
*Mx*

Things might be a mess, but there she was, still helping me. A true friend.

But still, Leroy appeared with greater intensity. I heard him laughing at me – taunting me.

I grabbed my keys and coat, determined to distract myself. In the supermarket, I figured I'd keep things simple, make the pounds stretch for as long as humanly possible.

I walked through the aisles in Tesco with an empty basket in hand, stopping to select a few vegetables from the fresh-produce aisle.

No sooner did I make my way down to the aisle of frozen food than I spotted the familiar outline of a man. I recognised his heft, those broad gym-built shoulders. Barry was in the aisle opposite, peering at the jars of olives and pickles, smiling cheerfully to himself as he grabbed a can of pulped tomatoes.

I walked over to him. 'Didn't think I'd bump into you in here,' I said stiffly. I figured he must be off duty.

Barry jumped back. 'Good grief! You gave me a fright. Do you always creep up on people like that?'

I rolled my eyes. I wasn't sure whether I trusted Barry

anymore. Someone had relayed to Barbara that I'd been uncomfortable treating Leroy, that I was incapable of being indiscriminate.

'Thought you'd be used to being jumped on,' I clipped.

He sighed, scratching his head. His attention moved swiftly to the next subject. 'I'm meant to be planning a meal for the missus, see. But shopping is taking ages. Reason why I never do it.'

I tutted, snatching the shopping list from his hand. He'd checked off basil, parmesan, olives. 'You're missing the main ingredient.'

'I don't suppose you know which type of pasta would work well?'

'Go for easy cook. Done in five minutes.'

Barry smiled. 'It's good to see you, Nina. How are you?'

'Up and down,' I sighed. 'A patient died on my watch because a gang member took priority. I imagine you've heard all about it.'

Barry paused, flummoxed, then lifted his basket from the floor. He grabbed my sleeve, leading me to the corner where I rested my back against a shelf.

'Look, I'm sorry,' he said. 'I heard what happened. But Dev's death wasn't your fault. There *were* other things you did which were questionable, however. It's best to accept the outcome and learn from it. We've got enough going on around here without a drama in Newgate as well.'

There was a fire in my chest. He had no clue what was really going on. Every time I heard his voice, his naïveté – justification for inaction, his blatant favouritism – I wanted to thump him.

'Who is he, Barry?'

I stared into his eyes, searching his pupils.

'What do you mean?' he asked.

'Why are the police so protective of him? He was there, that afternoon. I have the video. Why hasn't Leroy been arrested?'

Barry sighed, dropping his head. 'You're muddling the two. Firstly, it's not as easy as you think. There's a procedure to follow, it's based on evidence, which that video *isn't*. Secondly, he didn't hurt Balraj. I can tell you that.'

I rolled my eyes. 'They say Balraj will never walk again. Do you know that?'

Barry shook his head. 'That's not fair. I know you're worried about what's going on in Levinstone, but you're not the only one.'

'Should we expect another incident? Because I tell you, none of us feel safe. This is our home, but it feels like we're being forced out. What exactly are the police doing about it?'

Barry looked behind him to check if anyone was listening, then turned back. 'The police are working hard. Do you think it's easy – motivating – listening to everyone having a go at us all the time? Still, we've increased our presence. Doubled patrol efforts. We arrested at least five in the last month for public disturbance.'

'Well, I don't think it's working,' I said dismissively. 'And meanwhile, when they get into scraps, they strain whatever services we do have functioning in an already strained system.'

'I'm not being funny, but we all know you've got strange views about crime. Maybe you should retrain and join us if you feel so passionate about policing.'

I blinked.

'Now, if you don't mind,' he said, 'I need to get on. I'll see you at the next community meeting where we can continue this discussion.'

Barry grabbed his basket, walking down the aisle.

I called after him. 'I believe in karma, you know! What goes around comes around based on your deeds and actions.'

Barry waved goodbye, winking. 'We're working with Pastor Oswald Otis and Guru Shankar from the Shree Ram Hindu Temple and Community Centre. I think we've got karma covered!'

Walking up the narrow stairwell to my flat, I was thinking about Barry and Farah, wondering when she might respond. My hand had turned purple from where the handle of my shopping bag, hooked onto my wrist, had impeded my circulation. My hair was damp from rain.

I looked up, the carrier bag bumping against my thigh. To my surprise, I found Nikolaus outside my front door, ringing my doorbell. He turned when he heard the crinkle of plastic. Smiling, his face, his translucence, appeared as a ray of hope at the end of a very long day of struggle.

'I was thinking you were not at home,' he said.

'I went shopping.'

Breathless, I reached the top of the stairs and stood beside him, wiping my face in the crook of my elbow.

'Here, I help you.' He unhooked the bag from my wrist, and I clenched and unclenched my hand to get the blood flowing again.

Inside, we removed our coats. Nikolaus placed the shopping bag on the kitchen table.

I rushed into his arms, burying my face into his chest. He held me close, lifting my face, a finger placed under my chin. I wanted to surrender myself fully to him, to feel release from everything going on. Our lips met with an intense desire and forlorn longing. Hungrily, we peeled off our clothes, our tops, jeans, underpants, and clambered onto the sofa. We laughed deliriously when, in our enthusiasm, we knocked over a side lamp.

'Are you sure you want to?' he whispered.

I loved his strength and power; I kissed him hard. The evening melted as I wrapped my legs and arms around him. It was just what I needed, the comfort of his flesh, our bodies blending, moving in unison. Between us, an unspoken rhythm of understanding had emerged. I felt a rush of helplessness, a sinking yielding, a surging tide that left me weak. The night blurred and drowned into space as our bodies sank further into the cushions.

At first, his love was gentle and soft, then grew stronger, fiercer, as he exerted greater control.

Afterwards, we rested, quietly catching our breath. In the dark, our bodies were alive, skin damp yet electrified.

He stroked my limp hair as I placed a hand on his chest, easing my fingers through the fuzz to feel the thrum of his heartbeat.

'You are happy?' he asked.

I nodded, unable to speak. I didn't want him to see the tears rolling down my cheeks.

'I know what happened. Your friend, the curly-hair one

– she told me. What will you do now?'

I sighed. 'Look for something else, I guess. I've not been struck off. Just fired.'

I hoped I'd made that clear to Farah.

He was silent. 'You are smart and beautiful. You will find something.' He kissed my forehead, but I felt a heaviness take over me. Nursing at Newgate was all I knew. Despite Nikolaus here, the weight of the injustice I'd endured rained down heavily.

'I'm keeping positive,' I said, but by now he was drifting off to sleep, his breathing slow, and after a few minutes, the faint sound of his snoring.

Gently, I peeled myself from his arms, creeping quietly to the kitchen. I was thirsty for water, and I sat down at the kitchen table and lit a candle. Watching the flame flicker and dance, I grabbed a pen and pad of paper. I began writing:

*I'll probably live with the guilt for the rest of my life. If there's anything I could do to change what happened, believe me I would. Though good things are happening, wonderful, positive things, how can I forget what I did? I feel like I can't move on until a score is settled. I'm growing obsessed by it.*

I heard Manisha's voice in my ear: *You* – you *are responsible, do you know that?* You *neglected my son. What – or* who *– was so important that you could not keep an eye on him?*

I closed my eyes, contemplating how nothing in life is for free, certainly not healthcare in the United Kingdom, nothing I needed and wanted to live. But I had the power to choose who I loved, the power to choose between right and wrong.

I pulled out the drawer from under the kitchen counter and stared at the box of morphine I'd stolen from Newgate. The tablets rattled in the crinkly plastic between my fingers as I prised them out of the silver strips. Pop, pop, pop went the purple tablets in the centre of my palm. Walking to the toilet, I dropped them into the basin.

On my return, I picked up my phone. It was then that I saw what Farah had done.

*Levinstone Gazette*
*Saturday 5th November 2022*

*NURSE FIRED FROM NEWGATE HOSPITAL*
*Investigation into patient's death exposes severe failures in patient care.*

*Senior Nurse Nina Dabral has been fired for 'serious failures in nursing duties'. This included essential medication discrepancies, inadequate note-taking, even displays of hostile and antagonistic behaviour towards patients. These were the findings from an investigation into the death of patient Dev Shah, a talented twenty-year-old singer-songwriter, admitted at Newgate with a case of suspected appendicitis. Though Nina's actions were not found to have contributed to Dev's death, it is suggested that his quality of care was severely compromised during his final hours.*

*This is just one instance of what staff at Newgate Hospital have called chronic failings in patient care.*

*According to one source, financial pressures have caused management officials to take drastic action. Operational spend has been cut including investment in staff required to take care of increased numbers of patients. This has led to poor patient care, which left unchecked and unreported for long durations has caused Newgate to be fined for missing key NHS targets. 'It's a vicious cycle,' said one source. 'Patients are now at serious risk.'*

*One staff member said about Mr Shah's death: 'The issue remains, there was not enough staff available to check on what Nina was doing. A serious lack of investment has intentional as well as unintentional consequences.'*

*Another source close to the hospital said: 'Nina's case highlights the problem that exists. We have a right to know why all manner of issues at Newgate have not been brought to light sooner, with necessary action taken. How many more patients must die before something changes?'*

*The* Levinstone Gazette *is calling for a public inquiry.*

*Do you or someone you know work in Newgate Hospital? Reach out to speak to us in confidence at: Farah_First@LevinstoneGazette.com*

# 24

I parked my car, waiting for Farah under the bridge. In my rear-view mirror, I saw her white VW Polo pull up behind me in front of the recycling bins. She switched off her lights and glanced sheepishly at me.

*Keep calm, just breathe. I am loving and kind, not at all aggressive.* I squeezed my keys tightly in my hand.

I climbed into Farah's car, lips pursed. Farah remained silent.

'So—' I stared straight ahead, determined to contain my outrage. I watched a man climb out of a van in front, fly-tipping a soiled mattress.

'Want to tell me how that article happened?'

She turned away. 'Nina, I can explain—'

I stared at her smug profile, wanting to punch her face.

'I gave you information proving corruption at Newgate – you said it was your responsibility to report to the public. But still, you landed me in the shit. Naming and shaming me for something I did not do.'

'Nina, please calm down.'

She had a bloody nerve. 'Dev's death was not my fault.'

'Okay, just hear me out.' Farah glanced to the side, watching a man with a dog walk by. 'I wanted to protect you, to keep your name out of it,' she said. 'But my editor . . .'

'What about your editor?' I snapped. 'Those emails were exposing. Why didn't you use them?'

She sighed as if already worn down by our conversation. 'I couldn't, okay?'

'But why? It makes no sense!'

'We have to be careful since . . . everybody is connected somehow.'

I swallowed. 'What are you saying, exactly?'

'My editor . . . he knows Richard. The matter is *sensitive*. Besides, he wanted a live case, to drive home how serious the failings in Newgate are more generally, not to make it personal.'

'Personal? Personal to whom exactly?'

'Richard.'

'What about *me*, or do I not matter?'

'It needed to be this way, to justify the call for a public inquiry, which is a big ask. Readers want a human angle. So, we needed to give them . . .'

'Thanks,' I hissed.

She fell silent. 'You were let go, Nina. And for good reason.'

I leaned my elbow on the window's edge, a hand holding up my heavy head.

'You realise you're protecting Richard, so he can continue hiring his relatives, profiting from carrying out endless blood tests. That decision is bad enough, but on top of it, innocent workers will lose their jobs. Don't you get it?'

'They let you go after a patient *died*. It was relevant, and central to the story of healthcare provision. It's in the public's interest to know about it. I did warn you it might happen.'

'You said you'd protect me if I gave you something bigger.' My throat felt dry and hurt from raising my voice. 'I gave you something bigger. This is huge!'

'But you also know, those other things they let you go for were serious.'

I bit my tongue.

'I'm a journalist, alright?' she said.

'Like I don't know that.'

'I love my job just as much as you love yours. But there are games I must play.'

'I've lost my job,' I said.

'I'm sorry. Really, I am.' Though from the way she said it, it was debatable. 'It's unfortunate the story landed like that. It's not what I wanted.'

'Unfortunate,' I said. '*Unfortunate* is that you've made me out to be a negligent nurse. You know as well as I do, there are so many questions left unanswered. But, oh no, you take a swipe at me. Write me off. Mixing me up with the other horror stories going inside Newgate. Failing to use vital pieces of information I sent you – which I risked my own safety and freedom getting.'

She writhed uncomfortably in her seat. 'We should probably talk about how you obtained that information.'

'I need another job,' I said, ignoring her. 'How am I supposed to get one now when my name is in print?'

It irritated me to see Farah tapping her thumb on the steering wheel.

She appeared to be turning something over in her mind. 'Look, I'm sorry, okay? I tried to write the story we both wanted . . . but I—' She clenched her jaw. 'I probably shouldn't be telling you this, but . . .'

I sat back. 'What now?'

'Dev's mother . . .'

I was taken aback. 'Manisha?'

Farah nodded.

'What about her?' Most likely this was one of Farah's story-dealing distraction techniques. I thought I should be careful and not fall for it.

'She doesn't accept the findings of the internal investigation nor the coroner's verdict. She's got lawyers – good ones. A guy called Sid Waqar who is known to be ruthless. Let's just say . . . I know him well. He's advised her that something doesn't add up. There's no way her son could have died of something natural.' Farah's look was intense.

'And?'

'She's calling for an independent investigation. If the hospital is covering something up, an independent investigation will expose it. I will certainly be reporting on it.'

'Or it will cause further problems for me,' I said, 'because I already know what's going on. A conflict of interest with MediCentral. You know, it's ironic that with so many blood tests carried out on Dev, they found nothing.'

I thought of the morphine, too. How stories about me were most likely swarming like flies around a sewer. 'It's over for me,' I said. 'They've fired me. So, what happens now about Dev, or his death – or even MediCentral – doesn't change things.'

'Something might come out that could help clear your name,' she said. 'Just thought you'd want to hear that, to give you some hope.'

I snorted. I knew Farah's game. She still wanted me as a source, hooked in on false promises. She was no better than the drug dealers on the streets. But her poison was stories that led to yet more stories, regardless of the consequences.

'My job is to be objective,' she continued, 'to see it from the perspective of the public. I'll be in touch with anything relevant, I promise. I just need more time.' She pulled out her vape and sucked hard on the end, releasing a long, smoky, white trail.

'I'm not sure if I trust what you say anymore,' I mumbled. 'I'm not sure if I trust anyone.'

I was now thinking of Nikolaus. Why I'd ever been stupid enough to think this relationship would be any different to the countless others I'd had and failed at. He was too good to be true. Any minute now, he'd see my true colours.

'Regardless of what you might think, what I did was for the greater good,' Farah said.

And there it was, her self-delusion.

I shook my head and climbed out of her car, just as the man fly-tipping the dirty mattress drove off in his van.

# 25

The air in my flat was stale. The room around me appeared smaller and strangely tilted. I was convinced that, if I closed my eyes, the walls would tremor and inch forward. I'd been rereading Farah's article, repeatedly, as a way of torturing myself. And while the article did not implicate me in Dev's death, it had ruined my good reputation as a nurse. I didn't think I would ever come back from it.

I drank whatever I could find. A half-bottle of gin. A few shots of cheap whiskey. As the alcohol mixed, I no longer cared what I did. I began detaching from my thoughts, the overwhelming burden of responsibility.

The alcohol set my throat aflame. Pain and pleasure merged to become one.

I pulled out my phone and sent Mercedes a text:

*Love yo9ux!! Tank you for the m8ney & 4 Evy thing! X*

She messaged back:

*Don't ever mention it. You don't deserve what happened! Text you later! x*

I had intended to sleep, to wake up the next day hung-over, with every bad thought obliterated. But as I lay flat on my back, my mind still turning, I needed fresh air. I had to get out.

I grabbed my keys, my coat and phone, and headed to the local park. I thought nothing of it at the time. With every staggered step, I was sinking into a pit. One filled with quicksand, legs submerging, the air around me pulling me in.

In Levinstone Park, I passed oak trees on my left, a football pitch to my right. A little boy wearing a blue-and-white T-shirt dribbled a ball across the grass. I saw him kick it into a goalpost. His mother jumped to cheer him on. That open display of affection, mother to child, made me want to hurt myself.

I found a bench in front of a pond, the water filmed with grey, and I gazed out through the mist. I sat down to catch my breath, to contemplate everything that had happened. Dev's death. Manisha's approach. Being fired – this hideous story now in the papers. A flock of pigeons arrived at my feet. Bobbing heads, scavenging for food, they pecked at the remains of a mouldy sandwich.

I kept reminding myself that I was never wanted, so nothing that came next should be at all surprising. My parents were the first to abandon me, my hospital family the latest.

My life was such a mess. How could I ever make sense of it. Maybe I hadn't been left in a basket after all. Maybe I'd been wrong, that the depressing episode of my early life was simply something I'd made up. Or perhaps it did happen, but it was a spiritual test, manufactured by the gods, to help strengthen my resolve to become a more empathetic person. Maybe being a nurse, losing my job, was part of that test. I needed to better learn how to offer selfless service to others.

Or maybe . . . my parents were in a forbidden relationship. My mother fell pregnant with no way of introducing me to his or her parents. Perhaps they were too strict or highly religious. She did what any young woman would do in an otherwise impossible situation. My mother was certain I'd be found. After all, she'd left me, not just in an ordinary place, like on a church or hospital doorstep, but in an important place: the nucleus of Great British political power.

Or . . . perhaps my mother was alive, and my father was dead. Or my father was alive, and my mother ran away. Either way, neither parent ever intended any harm. They just couldn't look after me, that was all.

But then, there was an alternative explanation for my existence too, one that implied I was a mistake. Unwanted. A downright nuisance. Born of a terrible crime, perhaps a rape in a back alley, or from sexual abuse.

I preferred not to think about that last option; I preferred not to know. It was why, all these years, I'd never allowed myself to become consumed with the silly notion of finding my parents.

The dark voice inside my head, the one I'd previously managed to contain, came forth stronger, more bitter, twisted, and judgemental. Sodden with alcohol, it told me, repeatedly, how I was destined to be alone, abandoned. A fuck-up for the rest of my life, no matter how hard I tried to do well. Of all the options I'd considered, it boiled down to this: I was abandoned at birth because, in the end, that was more favourable than my own mother looking after me as any loving mother would.

Had I enough strength to fight this voice off, to overpower it, to wrestle it to the ground with the dominance of my own truth and a glimmer of hope, I would have.

But broken as I was, that negative voice grew stronger and louder.

I hauled myself up, passing the pitch, staggering along the crooked path circling to the other side of the green. Mothers pushed prams, peering over their snug babies swaddled in creamy cellular blankets. A jogger ran past glancing at his watch. Toddlers skipped freely, oblivious to how lucky they were to have their parents close.

I was breathless, my body weak. I stopped at a bench, just in front of the play area with log-framed slides, swings, a mini roundabout graffitied with the letters *SKillaz*. I scanned those letters now drizzled with rain. I unfolded a plastic carrier bag from my pocket, placing it flat onto the damp seat covered in bird droppings.

The sun cast a dusky glow over the expanse of muggy green. Something in the distance caught my eye and I straightened.

A group of young men, silhouette outlines, appeared in front of me. Nearing, I saw they were wearing black tracksuits and fluorescent white trainers. My throat constricted, watching them stride with the street swagger and confidence the rest of us lacked, their arrogance that of a ruling clan. They drew closer as one.

Fear hooked into my stomach as I remembered that scene from the bus, the carnage caused by groups like these. Just like in my dream, I found I couldn't move. Around me, people grew agitated, searching for an escape route.

Mothers grabbed their children's hands. Bikes, tricycles, prams pushed in a frenzy at high speed. People walked, then ran, towards the park exit.

One of the men was walking like a shadow at the front of the crowd, limping, then pulling away from them. He stopped after a few steps in front of a chestnut tree, and stood hunched like an old man short of breath. He pressed his hand onto his stomach and pulled out his phone, placing it to his ear. It was the simple gesture of him glancing around, left to right, that made me realise who it was.

Leroy.

My body trembled.

I should have left right then, knowing what he was capable of. I'd seen him attack Balraj. I needed to get out of the park before he spotted me. But we shared an unspoken connection, a frequency, a moment of life and death now swollen into something greater than just the two of us. It might seem nonsensical to others, but to those involved – one cared for, the other, carer – the umbilical healthcare cord connecting us was thick like hanging rope.

I felt compelled to listen in on his conversation. He must have read my thoughts because he looked up. I moved my face away quickly, walking towards a cluster of trees. All the hatred inside me welling up.

He sensed my presence, and ended the call. Then stared at me piercingly as the world around us receded. Recognition descended and his expression fell, curving into a malevolent grin.

'Oi, you! You, that *nurse*! Bad nurse, Nina, hold up!'

My heart jumped into my throat. My head rushed from the slosh of alcohol. I averted my eyes and began walking towards the park entrance. I dared not turn. Behind me, I heard him laugh.

'It *is* you. I knew it!'

It was too late. His feet swished in the grass as he picked up speed, and he trotted to the side of me, his strength and dynamism returned. I marched on.

'Oi, killer nurse, you not working now, are you?'

'Go away, Leroy.'

My eyes remained fixed on the concrete ground, scanning the grey, blurry stone. A few more metres, and then I'd be out. I could shake him off easily on the main road.

'Hold up!'

He was panting like a dog on a hot summer's day.

'Did you do it? Did you kill that man?' he said. 'I just want to know because, I swear, I *knew* there was something wrong with you.'

I stopped, staring at him, his eyes strangely alive, pupils wild and dancing. Shadowed in dark circles as they were, I sensed a flash of sadness.

'What exactly do you want?' I asked.

He laughed once more, sneering, taunting me.

I walked away, telling myself I was not there to rise to his insults. Baseless. Lacking in substance.

Fucking Farah. And as for Leroy. Well. We all knew what *he* was.

'You come over all high and mighty but look at you now!' he said. 'No different to me. You're fuckin' careless, from what I hear.'

Out of nowhere, his accomplices gathered around him, but he shouted for them to keep back. He had this one covered, he said. 'We ain't gonna shook her. She's safe. That's Nina, killer nurse. Her story was in the papers!'

They roared with laughter, excited by meeting me, an unlikely local celebrity.

'You don't know anything about me!' I called, my voice trailing. I kept walking, thinking I'd finally left him behind. I was nearly there – at the park gates. But Leroy was behind me, determined to continue.

'But that's where you're wrong, see,' he said, struggling to keep up. 'I should fucking kill you for creeping up on me that night. You think you're better than me. But look at you now. Look who's the criminal!'

He moved to my left. I noticed his bracelet, his wrist exposed. His arm jittered around his stomach. Around his neck, a thick rope – gold, with a crucifix dangling.

'They had to get rid of you,' he said, staggering. 'That's how bad you are. Want me to find you a job? We could do with a nurse in our group . . . we like psychopaths.' He laughed and coughed, all at once.

My thoughts rushed and sloshed around. I didn't need this right now. I needed to get out. 'I'm nothing like you,' I hissed. 'You go around stabbing people in gangs. *I* don't do that.'

'You think you know what you saw. And based on that, you're passin' judgement. But trust me, you don't know jackshit about that night, so just stay out of my business.'

The group of men were to my right. One of the men wore sunglasses, a red scarf. He smoked the last of a joint, then threw the stub into the grass. He stopped, stamping his foot as Leroy called out to the others.

'Later, yeah?'

The man in the sunglasses nodded. The rest of them swiftly dispersed, moving behind and around me, overtaking me as I deliberately slipped back. It seemed whatever they had planned wasn't happening now, so I got out of their way, allowing them to slip towards the car park. They clambered onto their bikes, seven or eight, all lined up beside the gate.

'That's the trouble with people like you. Holier-than-thou,' Leroy said.

Now he was alone and less of a threat, I stopped and turned around. 'What did you say?'

'At least I accept what I am. Who the fuck are *you*? That's what I can't figure out.'

The anger inside made my body hot and feverish. A flock of pigeons circled overhead, squawking, moving towards the pond, then heading back towards us again. Like tossed paper in the breeze, grey and white, they were turbulent, unrelenting.

'You're an imposter, impersonating good,' he said, 'but anyone who gets a kick out of manipulating the sick has got to be sick herself!'

My fury was far deeper than just this one man, but now he was the embodiment of everything I hated and resented in this town. I wanted him dead. An innocent man had died and here *he* was, carrying on with his life.

I walked away. Leroy seemed resigned to let me go, but not before firing one final shot.

'I can give you something . . . to take the edge off the pain. Any time you want, Nina. Hope to see you again.'

I turned, lunging forward, my hand mid-air, fist clenched tight. But I restrained myself. I was not that kind of person. Leroy laughed, a full belly laugh, throwing his head back, bending forward – crying even.

'Oh God! I shouldn't do that. My stomach!'

The wind carried his laughter further. I walked faster to the park's entrance, the air growing darker around me.

As I walked out, turning right down the street, I debated whether to call Nikolaus. But my battery power was ten per cent. Mercedes had sent a text:

*Are you okay? Been drinking? LOL! Your last text! SERIOUSLY!! Had to reread it. You go for it, babe. Go celebrate. Despite them mentioning your name, everyone is talking about Newgate! It's what you wanted. Will pop round when I can. xxx*

The street was empty and quiet. Behind me, a car engine drew closer. A boxy black Mercedes G-Class with blacked-out windows flashed past me towards the park.

I peered back at the park through the metal railings. The hum of the engine quietened. I couldn't quite see the car or where it was positioned. But I heard tyres crunching against the tarmac, and caught the light from two headlights moving in the distance. Yellow orbs glowed in an opening to a cluster of green. I could just about make out a lone figure emerging from a bush. From his limp and walk, I knew it was Leroy.

The engine of the G-Class cut out. A clink and tinker of metal as the engine cooled down. A man emerged from the vehicle and shuffled onto the grass, his body thick, his feet trudging.

Leroy lit up a cigarette. Ribbons of smoke wafted in the slight wind. He nodded to the man and continued scrolling through his phone.

I slipped back into the park, skimming over the grass. I found another tree to hide behind, close enough so I could hear them talking.

I could tell the other man was Barry, just from the manner of their conversation.

'Why are we meeting here? This is fucking dangerous,' Leroy said.

Barry replied, 'We had a deal. You don't get to call the shots.'

'I said I'm not dancing to your tune, yeah? I ain't changing my mind, either. You lot are all the same, thinking about yourselves. No consideration of the risks I'm taking.'

Barry's voice hardened. 'You don't seem to understand how serious this is.'

'I can't wait any longer,' said Leroy. 'I need to get out – you don't seem to understand. I'm losing myself!' I wondered how this connected to the conversation I'd overheard in the ward. Here, Barry was not so fatherly. He waved his hands about. Still, what a cheek, those bloody two. Conspiring to work together when innocent people in the local community, ones who worked hard for a living, were left exposed without protection. Balraj had been stabbed.

My body wound up tight like a screw.

Barry turned, walking to his car. 'You need to hurry up!' he called. 'We need this over.'

'You still don't get it,' spat Leroy. 'I should never have been left hanging for this long!'

Barry climbed into the driver's seat. I heard the door clunk, the engine starting. The car accelerated immediately and performed a sharp U-turn. I saw his arm bend as he turned the steering wheel. Tyres squelched in the muddy grass. Without even a sideways glance, he zoomed out of the park.

Leroy stood there, white jogging bottoms ruffling in the breeze. I remember a glint of light illuminating the side of him. He was on his phone, frantically typing.

In the distance, I heard the approach of another car.

At first, I thought it was my imagination playing tricks on me. Or that, perhaps, Barry had returned because he'd forgotten something. The engine roared louder, angrier. I saw the car flash past towards the entrance. This one looked like a black Ford Ranger. Then, out of nowhere, I heard a volley of gunshots. My ears rang from the noise, the air throbbed from the vibration.

My stomach clenched; I was holding my breath. I heard a man yell 'fucking snitch'; tyres screeched as the car reversed and zoomed out. The windows were wound down. Howls and shrieks of wild laughter trailed the air like animals dragged back into the horror-filled darkness.

*What the fuck?!*

In the park, Leroy staggered; his body halted. He collapsed, falling onto his stomach in a patch covered in bark chips. His left leg juddered; his right arm strained forward. He reached out for something beside him, clawing at the grass, but then . . . he was still.

I heard the blood rushing in my ears, the adrenalin firing in my veins. The sounds around me, the rustle of leaves, flies buzzing, the flapping of moths' wings, now all so acute. In this electric moment of violence, my senses had heightened. I waited, unable to move, unsure whether it was safe to approach Leroy. Eventually, I leaned over him. He groaned, and my mind scrabbled for clarity on what I should do next.

'Are you okay?' I said.

His eyes rolled and darted around as if trying to process what just happened. 'I w-w-won't . . . make it.'

I kneeled over him, observing the blood seeping from his stomach, his gasps sudden and irregular. His hands twitched and crossed over him. 'C-call m-my mum . . .'

'You need an ambulance. Just hang in there,' I said.

His legs jerked. He sucked the air in and out of his lungs as if breathing through a straw. He nodded, but only just.

'You'll be fine – do you hear me? You'll be fine!' It was a desperate attempt to sound calm. But inside I was panicked. I staggered back, peeling my arms out of my jacket. I mopped up the blood gushing from his stomach and pressed down hard with the back section of the material. My fingers were stiff and cold, but my shoulders felt hot and burned. Leroy cried out in pain, releasing a *ha-ha-ha-ah* sound as I worked to stabilise him.

'Wh-h-at the fuck . . .?' he said, his breaths light, a whisper. 'G-grace . . . c-call her.'

'I'm saving your life,' I snapped.

Even with him in that state, Leroy managed to judge me. This man was really something, I thought. Why had I bothered to help him? No longer was I employed as a nurse. I had no obligation whatsoever to be there for him. It was natural for him to want his mother, but right now, he needed medical professionals.

I peered down at him. 'Where's your phone?'

He did not answer. His eyes remained closed.

'Leroy! Can you hear me? Where is your phone?'

I looked around him, searching for his phone. I spotted it just to the side of him and grabbed it, intending to make the call to emergency services and leave him shortly after.

'I need your pin,' I said, cold, matter of fact.

'Seven . . . Nine . . . Four . . . Seven . . . Seven . . . Nine . . .'

Just saying those numbers took considerable effort. I stared at the outline of him, knowing his wounds were too deep. After the stabbing he'd sustained, now the gunshots, his condition was critical.

'I'm calling the ambulance now,' I said. 'Just hang in there.'

Here I was, desperate to get him seen, when all this time I had resented his priority treatment.

He coughed and spluttered; his eyes closed once more.

'I c-can't be left. They will . . . k-kill me . . .' he spluttered. How had he known I'd intended to call the ambulance and then leave him there, alone?

It was possible Leroy might survive this, but chances were slim. If he did, I knew the quality of his life would most certainly be diminished. He might never walk or eat as normal. With what had happened to Balraj, that prospect felt like poetic justice.

I managed to dial 999, the phone slippery from the blood. They picked up after three rings.

'Emergency services. Which service do you require?'

I closed my eyes, my heart racing. I pressed the phone close to my ear, placing a hand over the mouthpiece. 'Ambulance. A man is shot. He's dying. You need to come fast!'

'Please hold.'

I glanced behind me to ensure no one was there. I stared down at Leroy, who by now was making gurgling sounds.

The operator returned.

'How can I help?'

'I've already told you. I need an ambulance!'

'Where is the patient now? Are you with him?'

'He's in a park – in Levinstone.'

'Is he breathing?'

'Yes, but he's struggling. His injuries are too severe. He has sustained a gunshot wound to the abdominal region. Entry wound – left midclavicular line of the abdomen. Circumferential appearance, about one centimetre in length. Exit wound – I can't see, it's too dark. Possible vascular trauma – I can't stop the bleeding!'

'We'll get there as quickly as possible. We are contacting the next available vehicle.'

I was silent.

'Madam, are you still there?'

I hesitated. I knew what that meant. From the last few briefings I'd had in Newgate they'd told us that waiting times were well over an hour.

'Ma'am, are you a medical professional? Can you confirm your exact location?' She spoke slowly, carefully, as I heard her fingers punch into a keyboard. 'Can you stay with him until the ambulance arrives?'

'We're in the park, by the thick cluster of trees.'

'And your name?'

My name . . .

'Ma'am. Are you there? Please tell me your name. Are you a medical professional?'

It occurred to me that I couldn't, or didn't want to, give them my name. Already they were asking too many questions – I'd said too much. Neither could I call Grace. Not after everything that had happened. I didn't want to become embroiled in this man's life. I wasn't currently a nurse. I wasn't obliged to help. I hung up.

I threw down the phone.

Around me, the silence in the park covered us like a blanket. I took a deep breath, feeling myself sinking into the mud and grass.

I stared down at Leroy. His eyes opened.

'W-what are . . . you doing? I-I need h-h-elp . . .'

I moved closer, watching him struggle for breath.

'You . . . don't like me . . . But *p-please.*'

'It's not that I don't like you, I despise you,' I said. I leaned forward, my face close to his. 'I hate everything you are, everything you did. I'm beginning to question what I'm doing here, to be perfectly honest.'

'You're . . . f-fucked up. . .' he said.

'Or maybe you've just gotten what you deserve.'

He stared at me, his eyes growing wider, ever more wild.

'Give me one good reason why I should spend any more time on you,' I said. 'Why I should have emergency services rush you into a hospital after what happened. Balraj. Dev. You seem to be the dark cloud hanging over us.'

'N-n-urse!'

'I see it now. I see it so clearly.'

He closed his eyes and swallowed, licking his lips. 'Why . . . are you like this?'

'Be quiet.'

'Y-you are a nurse . . . but y-you don't seem to want t-to take care of o-others . . .'

'You've brought all this on yourself. I should leave you to die.'

He fell silent. His eyes closing, flickering.

'I know you were left . . . that you were . . . not w-wanted . . .' he said.

I fell back, astounded. How did he know? Who gave him that information?

'B-big story . . . I research-ch-ched it.'

Something inside me burned. That's when I saw the metal glinting from the pocket of his jeans. I leaned forward, sliding the knife out, flicking it open. I held the blade up under the silver moonlight. So many had said that carrying a knife made it more likely you'd be stabbed. Stabbing Leroy with his own knife, I scoffed, would be so incredibly just.

He began jerking, kicking his legs. His eyes were wide, his breathing erratic.

'I-I'm not what you . . . th-th-ink,' he pleaded. 'D-don't d-do this . . .'

'I know who you are. I know what you did,' I said.

The blood splattered on my coat as I plunged his knife into his stomach. The movement was quick, clean – for sure, I did not see it as though I was killing him. This man had killed himself. This man had killed the spirit of others.

I sat beside him in the dark as the wind carried the silence.

# 26

Later, some said it was unfair to get Nikolaus involved. But at the time, it made sense. I certainly didn't have anyone else to call. It couldn't be Mercedes. There was no way she'd be able to shoulder this.

Leroy's eyes were open, vacant. I brushed my hands over his lids to close them.

I grabbed my phone, knowing I must stay calm. But I had five per cent battery left.

I dialled Nikolaus's number, moving away from Leroy, outside the orbit of any reflection of light.

Nikolaus answered after a few rings.

'Nina?'

I stood in silence. I was a shadow in the dark, floating like a ghost.

'I need your help,' I said. Hearing his voice, wholesome and real, brought home the severity of my actions.

'Are you okay? I know you are suffering. I am sorry, Nina. I read the article . . .'

'Please,' I said, cutting him off. 'I don't have much battery left.'

He paused. 'Sorry?'

'I need you to come. I'll explain everything.' My eyes welled; my chin wobbled. I bit onto my tongue to gain better control of my emotions.

'Okay, I come after work, by Uber . . .'

My heart thumped hard in my chest. 'No, Nikolaus. Can you be ready, like, now?'

He paused. 'What is happening, Nina? You are worrying me.'

I breathed harder, faster. I couldn't leave him like that. 'I've done something. I need to be able to trust you. If you don't want to know, or to get involved, just say so now.'

'What does it mean?' he said.

'A man is shot,' I blurted the words out.

Nikolaus fell silent, presumably stunned. In that state, and after hearing his gasp, there was no way I could tell him what I'd done to Leroy afterwards.

'I can't move him on my own,' I said. I felt the knife in my pocket, warm and wet with Leroy's blood.

I heard the rustle of papers, the scrape of a chair. I imagined Nikolaus at the front desk in the mortuary having bolted upright.

'But why you move him, I do not understand. Call the police, the ambulance. It is not your problem.'

'Nikolaus, he's dead. Please . . . I-I need your help.'

The chair must have fallen. I heard it crash.

'I can't leave him here because they'll trace me here. I can't be connected to *this* or to *him*. You've seen that article – you've seen what they're saying. I was in the wrong place at the wrong time, I *swear*. Please, it's urgent.'

'Okay, okay,' he said.

'I'll drive to Newgate,' I said, frantic, 'but then you must take the wheel . . .' I paused, swallowing. 'I've . . . had a bit to drink.'

He breathed heavily. 'Take a taxi, Nina. Do not—'

But I hung up. I took the knife out of my pocket and dropped Leroy's phone onto the tarmac. Stamping on it hard, smashing it into pieces, I took the biggest part from the broken pile, where I knew the SIM was lodged and, along with the knife, tossed it into the bin. I ran out of the park towards home. By the time I reached my car, parked behind the Samosa Hut, my lungs felt heavy in my chest.

I switched on the engine, aware something strange and surreal was unfolding. The roads were empty, the tyres screeched as I drove. I knew I needed to be careful to avoid the police pulling me over. I had blood on my hands. Only now, the full gravity of my actions, the terrible consequences, were sinking in. I'd stabbed Leroy – he was going to die anyway, but as sure as hell, I'd made sure of it.

I planned what Nikolaus and I would do. Firstly, destroy any evidence and remove Leroy's body. There was blood on the grass – that would need a wash. We'd need to make sure there was no clue as to what had happened.

I pulled up into Newgate Hospital, parking at the back entrance to the mortuary. I sent Nikolaus a text, hoping my battery would last. And after five minutes, he emerged from the exit, walking shiftily towards the car in a puffer with a giant furry collar.

I jumped out of my car, moving to the passenger side.

Nikolaus saw me and waved, running across the ramp, opening the driver's door. A rush of cold air sent a shiver down my back. He fell into his seat, turning to kiss me. For a second, I closed my eyes, disappearing into the warmth of him. A wash of relief and normality – a reminder even, that I was not a bad person.

'Are you hurt?' he said.

I shook my head, unable to say anything. He wrapped his arms around me, and I melted into him. As I pulled away, he stared down at the specks of blood on my top, his eyes widening at the sight of my reddened hands.

'I don't understand,' he said, the alarm visible in his face. 'Why so much . . . *blood*?'

'Nikolaus . . .'

He glared at me. 'What is happening, Nina?'

'I did everything I could to save him,' I said. 'I promise I'll tell you everything, but right now, we have to drive – we can't waste any more time.'

'But who are you talking about?'

'Leroy . . . a former patient of mine.'

Nikolaus stared at me, confused. But then, reluctantly, he turned the key in the ignition. 'And you are sure we must move him? I do not understand.'

'I never wanted to get you involved,' I said.

The last thing I wanted was to repeat the story in full. And yet Nikolaus deserved to know the truth. I owed him that – I owed him every intimate detail. I owed him so much more. I was falling in love with him, but under these circumstances, our love felt doomed.

As he drove, Nikolaus mumbled to himself in German. He glanced at me several times, his eyes wide and glaring.

I stared out of the window, the pavements golden under the light of the street lamps, wondering where I should begin. That familiar voice told me he'd surely abandon me.

His eyes were now fixed on the road ahead. Negotiating a little traffic, Nikolaus cleared his throat and shook his head. 'It does not make any sense, you understand, yes? You should leave him there if he is the man you say he is. A shooter, a killer. Leave the police to find him. You do nothing wrong, Nina.'

I knew I should be honest, but I couldn't tell him I'd stabbed Leroy when he was dying.

Sleepy terraces flashed by; I didn't know whether to laugh or cry.

'I went there to get some air after a few drinks. Leroy showed up, then Barry. They were arguing, and then it . . . happened. He wouldn't have made it, Nikolaus. He was dying . . .'

Nikolaus accelerated as we passed a chicken shop. I realised, when seeing the vibrant logo, red, yellow and white, just how hungry I was.

'And then?'

I felt my body sway, my weight thrown to one side as Nikolaus steered left.

'Tell me, I need to know the truth,' he said, 'if I am to help you.'

He drove the long way, cutting out the bridge and Mercedes' flat, heading towards the park from the opposite end of the route I'd taken earlier. I was relieved he'd taken control of the wheel. There was no way I could drive.

'What happened next is that . . . I heard the gang, or his own associates, calling him a snitch. I reckon he sold them out, talking to the police.' I felt my stomach clench. *Barry and Leroy – working together. Just not in the way I'd thought.*

'I suspect that's why he was shot in the first place,' I said. 'Can you believe it? All this time, the community problems have been about gangs. And there he was, high up and connected with law enforcement. He would never be punished for his crimes.'

'I see.'

'He hurt Balraj,' I said, my face burning. 'He permanently paralysed him but got away with it. Besides, taking him to the hospital, after all those bullets, would have been . . . unnecessary.' I pinched the skin on my hands. 'Newgate is already under-resourced. *Over an hour!* That's how long it would have taken the ambulance. There was every indication he'd sustained a traumatic injury with potential multi-organ damage. He would not have survived the waiting time. He was bleeding heavily.'

I sighed as we drove under a bridge, the scent of the damp bricks entering my nostrils.

'I resent it,' I said. 'I resent having to treat him. If anyone was responsible for everything that's happened, the looting, the stabbing of Balraj – *me* paying the price for losing Dev, it's him!'

Nikolaus was quiet, turning things over in his mind. 'Still, I do not understand why you stay there.'

'I'm a nurse; I couldn't just *leave* him.'

We were almost at the park. Nikolaus accelerated, driving faster past the shops. He turned into the side road and drove up towards the entrance. The street was lit up in orange and the road grew wider, emptier; dereliction became more pronounced as we neared its end.

We jumped over a pothole and my stomach flipped. A ramp to slow us down, and then the steel bars of the gate.

'An innocent man died because of Leroy,' I said. 'I did

what I had to – I had to leave him. I just want you to know that. Promise me you'll try to understand.'

I wasn't sure whether I was trying to convince Nikolaus or myself, but I was building up to a revelation, a confession of what had actually happened.

He lifted a hand from the wheel to scratch his head, then replaced it, steadying the vehicle.

We drove into the park, on the wide path down the side. I pointed. 'Just here. Cars aren't supposed to drive in, but this evening, they did.'

I sat upright in my seat, hearing the tyres crunch in the gravel. The wind whooshed outside the window.

Nikolaus slowed as we approached the clearing. He switched off the engine and lights. We climbed out of the car together.

The park was empty and quiet. For a second, I imagined Leroy might have got up and run off.

We walked faster, then ran to the spot where he'd fallen. It was a terrible nightmare, all this. Any minute now, I'd wake up and laugh. Maybe even note it down in my journal.

But Leroy was still there, just as I'd left him. I gazed down at his crooked outline, sprawled out in a bloody heap. I saw his head flopped to one side, a cheek pressed into the grass.

I heard crickets chirping in a nearby bush. I felt scared, suddenly, that someone might come out and shoot us.

We inched closer. Lifting my gaze to Nikolaus, I watched his gentle face.

'I need to tell you something,' I whispered. 'Please don't let that change anything . . . Promise me you'll try to understand.'

Nikolaus was breathing hard. He brought his face closer

to Leroy's and I stood next to him, a hand resting on his shoulder.

'Tell me,' he said as he fumbled for his phone, turning on the torch light. He shone the light onto Leroy's face, wincing as he streaked the phone across Leroy's stomach. The crucifix around Leroy's neck glistened in the moonlight. I reached for Nikolaus's hand and closed my eyes.

'I killed him.'

'What?'

Nikolaus pulled away, shaking his head. There were tears in his eyes as he placed a clenched fist to his lips. He bit hard on the knuckle.

'He was dying,' I said. 'I . . . had to – he was in pain and was dying.'

The silence in the night sky vibrated. Somewhere in the distance, I heard an owl hooting.

He staggered back, the torch light faced down, a hand swept over his stomach. 'Nina,' he said, struggling for breath. 'What are you saying?'

'I suppose you're worried you're involved,' I said quickly. 'But you can leave. It's fine. I'll call the police. I'll come clean about what happened.' I pressed my hands together, wringing them. 'It's okay,' I said. 'I totally get it. You don't have to implicate yourself. You never signed up to this. Forget you ever met me!'

My arms fell, dangling on either side of me. I stood breathless, searching his face for confirmation, even a sign, that he was okay with this.

'I'll be . . . fine,' I whispered. My lips were stiff from the cold; my body shivered.

He glanced up, searching my eyes, considering my offer to get out. But then, reaching out, he moved closer to me, stroking the side of my cheek, drawing his forehead to mine. He stared into my eyes up close; I felt his warm breath brush my nose, a profound understanding of our connection, our mutual abandonment.

'He is a bad man, and he deserved to die,' I said.

He took a deep breath and nodded. 'I will not leave you alone if this is something that was necessary to happen.'

I glanced up to the sky, and inside, I felt a wave of gratitude. 'Thank you,' I whispered.

He dropped his head, and within seconds, he sprang into action. His lack of hesitation is what I loved most about him; even now, his ability to transcend his emotions.

'We must think,' he said, his voice lower, dead serious. 'We must be careful.'

Nikolaus was a lot calmer than I thought he'd be. His composure was remarkable. He appeared assured, calculated and restrained, his bodily actions closely connected to his level-headedness.

We moved fast, lifting Leroy – me, grabbing his legs, Nikolaus, his arms. One, two, three, we hauled him into the back seat of the car. All the while, I held my breath as we struggled to straighten his body.

Leroy's position was awkward.

'Careful!' I said, as we moved his flopping head, his back carefully positioned against the backrest. 'Drive slowly, steadily. He's on his side – he could easily roll forward . . .'

'Where should we take him?' Nikolaus asked.

I looked up at the sky once more, watching dark clouds

float across the horizon. Silver light illuminated Leroy's face. He seemed almost angelic and peaceful.

'I have a plan,' I said. 'Get in the car.'

I checked the grass behind me, picking up the broken shards of plastic from the phone I'd smashed. Nikolaus was still standing there, watching me, disbelieving of the events now unfolding around him. There was blood – so much blood. I grabbed a bottle of water from the boot and emptied it over the grass. When I was done, I washed my hands, drying them on my bottoms. I tugged at Nikolaus's elbow, urging him to get into the car.

'Let's go,' I said.

The back door slammed, and we both jumped into our seats. We hurriedly belted up and Nikolaus pressed his foot onto the gas, reversing out of the green.

We drove steadily up the gravel path towards the exit. Tyres crunched into the gravel before meeting the smoothness of the tarmac. I let out an exhale as Nikolaus turned the wheel. A sense of relief was palpable even though the night was far from over.

'For sure, people will be looking for him – maybe the police, and the shooters,' Nikolaus said.

I turned to look at Leroy in the back and saw his eyes, the slits of white, a little open. His mouth hung to one side; I saw his ragged tongue.

We drove along the main road then turned left in the direction of Newgate Hospital.

'Wait,' I said, 'you need to turn around.'

Nikolaus blinked.

'We're taking him to the garage.'

# 27

Nikolaus was silent, his eyes darting between mine, the road, back to mine again. 'You mean we bring him . . . to my place?'

'You said the garage was empty, didn't you?'

He was speechless.

'It will give us time so we can work out what to do next.'

'But then what do we do? We cannot leave him there.'

'It's just for one night. We'll move him after that.' I needed time to think, but time, as I knew well, was a luxury in an emergency situation.

Even in death, Leroy was occupying undue attention.

Nikolaus clenched his jaw. 'We leave him in the hospital and maybe we also . . . leave. We get out from here. It is better. We cannot stay after this.'

I sighed. 'We can't run. It will look suspicious.'

Nikolaus was shaking his head.

'Stay calm and drive to the garage,' I said.

His eyes blinked fast, but soon, his breathing relaxed.

We drove along the main road, down Oldfield Lane, slowing down as Nikolaus negotiated the speed ramps. The heavy load on the back seat made us jump more than usual.

Nikolaus indicated right as we approached Screaming Motors. He wound down the window as if the atmosphere in the car was suffocating him. As we pulled up at the back of the garage, he switched off the engine. He took deep gulps of air, staring at Leroy in the rear-view mirror.

'Don't look,' I said.

Nikolaus got out of the car, slamming the door closed, not angry at me, but as I know now, scared for us both. I was dazed and confused by how suddenly the night had turned bleak. How a thick sheet of black had fallen onto both of us. I struggled to breathe, feeling like a foot was pressing down hard onto my chest. I watched as Nikolaus fumbled for his keys, unlocking the garage. He opened the shutters, motioning for me to pull in. The lights flicked on automatically as I entered.

Nikolaus let out a long exhale as I got out of the car and I heard him muttering to himself in German. He did this when he was stressed and overwhelmed, when he needed to think fast. If the circumstances were different, I might have found it adorable, watching him pace up and down on the black rubber floor, a hand pressed to his forehead, struggling with his English. But not like this. This was like a horror movie playing on TV. Knowing it was my fault that Nikolaus was feeling increasingly unhinged, I thought it best to give him a few minutes.

After a while, I crept out of the car and stared at Leroy's body through the back passenger window.

Leroy appeared still, peaceful, his body limp, his mouth and eyes now fully open. I stepped back, unable to look at him anymore, his sweatshirt covered in blood. I staggered to the old couch, crashing onto the sofa where the cushion sagged. The wooden slat hit my tail bone, and I covered my face with my hands.

'This is bad,' Nikolaus said. 'Very, very bad.'

He removed his jacket, throwing it to the side of me, complaining it was feeling heavy. He pulled at his collar, his brow perspiring. Patches of yellow sweat were visible on the underarms of his white T-shirt.

My body felt empty and numb. We were both so deep in it now.

'We need to think carefully about what to do next. If anything goes wrong, we could be thrown in jail.'

I closed my eyes.

'For sure, you did not see the direction of the shooters?'

'What does that matter now?'

'What they say, exactly?'

'He is dead,' I said. 'Please, let's just focus on what we do next.'

I didn't know what to do with my body, my mind strangely alert and electric.

'Fuck!' Nikolaus shook his head. 'This situation is wild, Nina.' I could see what he was thinking, wondering if he'd been plucked from a more ordinary life and dropped, unaware, into this unfolding nightmare.

This would be the ultimate test of our relationship, I thought. I could not bear to think of him leaving me now. Of course, Nikolaus had already said he would stay, but the deeper the realisation of what I'd done, the more I began to question it.

What person in their right mind would do that for me?

Nikolaus continued to pace up and down, breathing heavily through his nose. 'Because Barry and Leroy know each other and have some arrangement, this means we have more problems.'

He was right of course. As overwhelm rushed over me, I experienced a sensation akin to drowning. I knew I must remain strong if Nikolaus was ever to survive this.

'I say we did the right thing bringing him here. His injuries were too severe,' I said. 'He would never have survived the shooting.'

'Maybe it is better you tell the truth. You were just there as a witness in the park, and you do what you think is right when he is dying. But you also . . .'

He covered his face.

Nikolaus held on to his chest as he struggled to breathe. He staggered to the couch, leaning an arm on the edge to better balance himself.

I felt my heart pounding as I threw myself into his arms.

'We will get through this, I promise,' I croaked. I was a survivor. I would not give up now.

We sat down and I held him tight, whispering in his ear how much I cared for him and wanted him in my life. I listened as he tapped his fingers on the armrest. Finally, he reached into his pocket and lit a cigarette. I watched as he blew out smoke, and with it, I heard him make a strange groaning sound.

'It does not change,' he said. 'I will be okay.'

'What doesn't change?'

He turned. 'My feelings for you.'

I swallowed.

'We are the same, you and me. I feel it that night. I still feel it now.'

I stared down at the floor; I felt a weight of responsibility for drawing this kind and innocent man into my crazy world.

'I could say the men got out of the car, and after shooting him, they stabbed him. I was there, and saw it all, and I panicked and called you – and you just followed what I asked.' I stared at him. 'That way, you can avoid trouble. I can say that we should have called the police, but I convinced you to go along with it. You could say you were traumatised, shocked. You didn't know what you were doing.'

Nikolaus nodded, like some of it was making sense.

'In a strange way, it's the truth. They can't prove I stabbed him.'

He nodded again.

But then it dawned on me. The knife. The phone. Why the hell had I thrown them into the bin? It all happened so fast. I hadn't been thinking properly.

'I need coffee. Do you want some coffee?' I asked.

'Okay,' he said softly, stubbing out his cigarette.

I got up and switched on the kettle next to a small fridge. The milk was spoiled; I poured it down the sink.

'We have to move him,' said Nikolaus. 'It is unlikely anyone will search for him, but for sure he cannot stay here. Patrick will return soon.'

'Patrick?'

'The owner of the garage. He returns in three days.'

My hand shook as I found two mugs. I spooned in sugar and then, from another tub, instant coffee granules.

'I've been thinking that we need to make sure there is no evidence of him left. He's in my car and I can't drive around with him in it.'

'We need some help. We cannot do it alone.'

I shook my head. 'The two of us is already enough.'

After a while, he said, 'Stefan could help us.'

I turned, hesitating, because the last thing we needed was more people involved in this. More people meant potential mistakes. Mistakes I could not afford to make.

'We are close. I trust him like I trust no other man. He is living in London. I know him since I was small.'

My face grew hot. There was a dead man in my car, yet here I was making coffee, discussing how to dispose of him. 'We can't tell anyone about this, we need to keep this contained!' A part of me was in denial, the other part, pragmatic.

Nikolaus moved closer, holding on to my waist.

'We'll find some woods – somewhere north of London, outside Lyndon Hill. We can dig a hole and bury him,' I said urgently. 'We'll work together. It will be faster.'

Nikolaus sighed.

'Teamwork!'

'But what if he is found by dogs?' said Nikolaus. 'They will search for him. It will be easy to find him. It is not good. We need another plan.'

'That *is* the plan. We dig deep and cover him with enough soil so you can't smell him. I'd prefer to burn the body but there would be too much smoke.'

Nikolaus pulled away, fumbling around for his jacket. 'You are a nurse. You know only of the living. I know the dead . . . I can help you take care of it, and also, Stefan.'

I felt a chill in the air as Nikolaus lit up another cigarette.

'Stefan is the right person to help.'

'I'm not sure—'

'He works in a crematorium.'

A strange feeling of relief swept over me.

I handed him a mug. 'Are you serious?'

'Very. He can be *trusted*, Nina.'

We fell silent, in reverence of the airy moment that swelled and contracted, a realisation descending, in the unspoken moments between us. We could not do this alone. Nikolaus was right. We needed an expert.

'You need to be sure there's no risk. We can't have something go wrong,' I said.

'Look at us, look at where we came from. The hardships we faced. They will say crime was inevitable, that we are . . . *damaged*.' He began pacing again. 'Stefan is like us. He had a hard life. He can remove the body, permanently.'

I flinched.

We moved to the sofa as Nikolaus stubbed out his cigarette. I leaned my weight onto him, resting my head on his shoulder. I closed my eyes as Nikolaus kissed my forehead, resting his cheek on my crown. I felt the warmth of his smoky breath bristle my hair.

And so, while every instinct of mine said to keep Stefan out, we had no choice but to bring him into the plan.

My head pounded from the alcohol and a wave of exhaustion hit me. Nikolaus placed his mug on the floor, got up and walked towards the car. 'It is the only way.'

I stood up and followed him.

'If you're sure.'

'There is no alternative.'

Nikolaus stopped and stared at Leroy through the window.

'We need to cover him for now,' I said. 'I can take care of things in the morning. I'll remove any last traces of evidence. As strange as it sounds, it's better he stays in the car for now.'

Nikolaus nodded.

'We need to call Stefan urgently,' I said.

'Of course.'

I moved closer, burying my face between his shoulder blades.

'There is carpet in the storeroom,' Nikolaus said. 'It's what we need.' He stroked my face reassuringly then walked towards the back. I traipsed behind him, my legs heavy. On the blue door a warning sign read: 'Authorised Personnel Only'.

Nikolaus pushed it open and switched on the light. The dust and smell of chemicals hit me in the face. I found it difficult to breathe, and covered my mouth with my sleeve.

He pointed to a rolled-up carpet propped in the corner. 'It is old. It was to be removed but I guess we use it now.' He walked towards it, prising the end of the scraggly rope wound around it. The roll of carpet slipped and toppled into his hands. He inched his fingers to the top while I rushed to grab onto the bottom.

We carried the roll out of the room, horizontal, negotiating the spare chairs, the narrow entrance. In the garage, I let my end drop to the floor. He untied the rope and kicked at the carpet; it fell open. It was stiff and hard, underlaid with sharp, piercing fibres.

We moved towards Leroy, then lifted him, one, two, three, out of the car, me grabbing his legs, Nikolaus slipping his hands just beneath his armpits. Leroy was beginning to grow stiff. With some relief, we dropped his body onto the edge of the carpet. Together, we rolled him four times. I had to stop after the second roll, to make sure Leroy's body remained straight, all the while thinking that perhaps things might just work out as planned.

We pressed down hard onto the edges, Nikolaus using the strength in his feet to roll Leroy's body securely with several kicks. I got to work, winding thick rope around what were once Leroy's moving ankles. Nikolaus moved to the top, repeating the action. I stared ahead, still picturing Leroy's face, that moment of shock when I'd stabbed him in the stomach as clear and visible as if it happened seconds earlier.

We hauled him up onto our shoulders like Indian villagers carrying a pail of water. My body trembled under the weight. I struggled to fish the car keys from Nikolaus's pocket. I opened the boot with one hand to stuff Leroy in. He just about fit. The car lowered under the weight of his dead body. Nikolaus slammed down the car boot securely.

My heart warmed watching Nikolaus move; with every passing moment, the two of us growing closer.

We both leaned our backs against the car, struggling to catch our breath.

After a while, we moved to the sofa and sat down. I scanned the smears of blood on the floor and noticed my hands. They were stained red. My head pounded as Nikolaus stood beside me, watching and listening.

'I must go to work to finish some things and then see Stefan. But I will call later, and tomorrow night we finish it.'

He moved towards me, kissing my cheek, offering me a spare key so I could come back to finalise arrangements as needed.

'No one will ever know he was here. I can clean up and leave everything sparkling.'

Nikolaus feigned a smile, but I saw the pain in his eyes. 'You will be alright? You call me, yes, if anything happens?'

I nodded, watching the garage door close behind him. Moving to the side, I turned up the heating.

I found blue overalls hanging on the wall and threw them on. I glanced around me, trying to figure out where I might start.

The pool of blood glistened on the floor. Smears from where the carpet had dragged, painting a bloody red path leading to the car.

Grabbing a handful of paper towels, I mopped up the blood, tossing them into a bin. My fingers moved quickly, purposefully, the muscle memory of nursing's speedy action still very much present. An innate instinct that, once learned, could never be erased.

I returned to the storeroom, delighting in the display of cleaning products and tools available. There were three kinds of mops, two brooms, a stack of towels, washing brushes. In a tub by the sink, a roll of steel wool and thick sponges. They were the kind used to wash cars; the kind most likely to be effective. Immediately, I thought of where I would begin, working furthest around where Leroy had lain, then moving closer to the vehicle. I'd need to mop the floor, then steam-clean it on full power using the electric steamer and its different-sized nozzles.

First, I stood silently for a while. It was just Leroy and me in the garage.

I returned to the boot and opened the door, slowly, staring

down at the roll of carpet. This man might have been dead, but in that moment, he felt very much alive. Lives had been forever changed by him. No amount of bleach enough to erase him.

'You realise, don't you, I tried to save you.' I talked down to the rug. 'I didn't expect you to die. That wasn't part of the plan . . .'

Blood was seeping through; I was aware the boot would probably need cleaning too.

'Who are you really, to be shot like that?'

The rug didn't move.

I slammed down the door to the boot, then moved to the side to find a roll of heavy-duty bags. I needed to discard anything that might have touched him, so I filled up a bucket with hot water and poured in bleach.

I began mopping up the remaining smears, intent on leaving the floor sparkling.

When I'd finished, the sweat dripping from my brow, I peeled off my gloves and threw them into the bin bag.

'I'm going now, but I'll be back,' I said as if Leroy might be listening. 'You understand, don't you, that we can't leave you here.'

But of course, he said nothing, neatly rolled as he was.

# 28

The next morning, I drove home early. The traffic was thick. The humdrum of life continued as normal. With the steering wheel weighing heavily in my hands, I couldn't take my mind off the thought that, in my boot, lay the body of a grown man.

But there was no way I could have risked leaving Leroy in the garage. What else could I have done but take him with me? I needed to get home and then return to the park. I couldn't do it now, however. Too many people about. I'd do it later, when it was dark. I'd remove the phone and knife from the trash can. I was overcome by a sense of frustration. My lack of intelligent thinking, in that critical moment, had made things so much more complicated.

As I drove, I thought about those conversations between Leroy and Barry. First in the hospital ward, then before the shooting. A sense of panic began to creep, because knowing that Leroy had a special arrangement with the police meant that, once they realised he was missing, he would be considered a priority missing person.

I gripped the wheel more tightly as I drove past the off-licence, partially boarded up from where looters, including Leroy, had smashed the windows that infamous weekend.

Spotting a free parking bay, I turned in, my body dictating an order for nicotine. It was something to take my mind off the escalation of events, the disaster looming.

A buzzer sounded as I opened the shop door. Lowering my face, I glanced to the side, scanning shelves floor to ceiling, eyeing bottles of wine, newspapers screaming headlines. I caught sight of a liquor stand, security cameras perched at each end of the shop. Like crows on the lookout for prey, they were a reminder of the growing possibility that I could easily be traced.

I covered my face.

Approaching the till, I slammed a twenty-pound note down onto the wooden counter. 'Twenty Camel Blue,' I said. Cigarettes cost more than food. I figured I had enough cans and sachets from the food bank to last me until at least Christmas.

A torso in a tank top opened the glass tobacco cabinet with a key. Even with his back turned, I knew it was Bernie Rogers. I recognised his ginger hair. His phone was wedged in his pocket at the back of his baggy jeans. His thick hands crinkled the plastic as he grabbed a packet of cigarettes from the top shelf.

He turned, peering at me.

'Nina, isn't it? I remember you; you came by the community meeting the other day.'

I swallowed and nodded, my mouth pressed into a lipless line. His was a question, or a statement, I couldn't be certain which.

He punched the price into the till, sliding the note off the counter with his index finger. 'You coming to the next one?'

I didn't want to talk. I didn't want a conversation about anything. I had a dead man in my boot. Just the thought of it was surreal, adjacent to this otherwise ordinary moment.

Bernie stared at me waiting for me to answer him.

'Maybe,' I mumbled.

'Looking forward to this next one. More focused, apparently.' He handed me the change, a pile of gold and silver in the centre of my palm. 'Restorative justice, Pastor Otis says. Should be entertaining.'

He smiled, staring down at the spread of papers as I averted my eyes.

'Terrible what's going on at Newgate, isn't it? They named you, I see. But I know it's not your fault. The way I see it, you did everything you could in an otherwise impossible situation. It's the bloody government. Thinking only short-term.' He glanced around his shop, boarded-up windows, shelves half stocked.

I was taken aback. His comments were unexpected and personal. 'A lighter, please.' I handed him a coin.

'Pressure's on at Newgate, now. Everyone's talking about it.'

I wished *he* would stop talking about it.

I stared at my feet, now feeling strangely disconnected from my ankles. Before he could say anything more, I scurried out of the shop and felt his eyes following me.

I returned to my car, waiting before getting in. I lit up a cigarette, clutching it like a novice with my thumb and forefinger. I thought of Leroy as he struggled to breathe in those final moments of his life. The thought of his body, now lifeless, curled up in the boot of my Nissan Micra.

I took a long drag of the cigarette, my hands trembling. I coughed and spluttered before finally exhaling.

What the hell was I doing?

I'd never imagined doing anything like this. No matter how bad my life had been, nor how difficult it was growing up, knowing deep down I wasn't wanted. No matter how bad it got at work – and Dev's death proved just how pressured it could be – I had always kept my cool, never letting it break me. But now, as I looked around me at the shops lining the road, falling signs, owners inside, desperate to keep business afloat, I was painfully aware of how I had snapped.

I grabbed my phone from my back pocket, checking my messages.

Nikolaus 10.30:
*All ok?*

Nina 10.30:

I drove to my flat, parking up in my usual spot at the back of the Samosa Hut. Climbing out, I pressed onto the lid of the boot to make sure it was securely closed.

Up the stairs to my front door, Mercedes was waiting for me on the landing. I glanced at her fishnet tights, slim ankles, black stiletto heels.

She turned when she heard me climbing.

'Had a good time, then?' She laughed, holding up a plastic bag. 'I got you a few bits. Wasn't sure whether you needed anything. Clearly, you've been busy.' She lifted her arm, the bag dangling. 'Bread, eggs, and pasta. Just wanted to make sure you were okay, you know, after that article landed.'

At the top of the stairs, I was breathless, my mouth dry and stale. 'I was out with Nikolaus. Not sure if I've mentioned him.'

Mercedes blinked. 'Thought so. He approached me looking for you. I told him what happened, and he seemed very concerned. Didn't realise you two were—'

I fumbled around for my keys, the jagged edges cold and sharp against my skin. 'I never got a chance to tell you the latest, not with everything going on.' I unlocked the door and pushed it open with my hip.

I could almost hear Mercedes' thoughts. *I can't believe you two got together. Why didn't you say? I knew he'd chatted you up in the pub . . . but you never said things escalated!*

'How long has it been going on?' she asked.

Inside my flat, the walls appeared thicker, moving, like any minute now one would capsize, crushing me to death.

I peeled off my top, catching sight of my sunken face in the mirror. Bloodshot eyes, beads of sweat. There was even a smear of red on the side of my left cheek.

I wiped it away quickly with my finger.

'You look terrible.' Mercedes peered at me. 'You've been drinking, haven't you? That text you sent was hilarious. Where were you, on some sort of bender? Just look at your shirt – smeared with ketchup!'

I washed my face in the kitchen sink, then ran into the bathroom to change.

I emerged, moving to the sofa, collapsing into a giant cushion.

'I'll make us tea, then, shall I?' Mercedes busied herself in the kitchen, placing the bread on the counter, eggs in the fridge. She was quiet for a while, as if figuring out what to say next. I felt a strange vibe, like a distance had grown between us.

'So how have things been with you? Any more news from that journalist?'

'I confronted her,' I said, 'after the story came out. Asked her if that really was the best she could write. But you know what they're like, cherry-picking what's useful. There's a connection, it seems, with her editor. So her story was heavily curated.'

She turned. 'Connection?'

'Editor knows Richard.'

'Jesus. What now?'

'Now, nothing. I get on with my life. Look for a new job or go on the dole.' I bit my lip.

Mercedes was quiet for a while. 'And Nikolaus?'

'What about him?'

'I heard he works in the mortuary . . .'

I detected a hint of judgement. 'It's temporary,' I said.

Mercedes leaned over the counter, clasping her hands. 'Not being funny, Nina, but isn't that a bit . . .'

I shot her a look. 'A bit what, exactly?'

'Morbid. Nina. A bit. *Morbid.*'

'It doesn't bother me. Why does it bother you?'

She turned, filling the kettle. 'I'm being judgemental,' she said, switching it on, 'but how do you know he hasn't killed someone?'

My stomach twisted.

'He's kind, and . . . dependable. We have a strong connection.'

I saw a flash of Nikolaus driving last night, that sight of him biting hard into his knuckle.

Mercedes returned to the counter. 'That night in the pub must have been some night.' She laughed.

I lay on my back. Closing my eyes, I listened to her clanging dishes. 'Yeah,' I said. 'It was.'

'Well. You'll never guess the developments at Newgate after the story came out.'

My eyes opened.

'Loads of closed-door meetings, that's what. I figured it must be with the Care Quality Commission. Bad timing, and all that, what with the prospect of the nursing strike happening.'

I sat up.

Mercedes watched me with arched eyebrows. 'It's a PR crisis for them. We've all voted to strike, standing with the Royal College of Nursing. According to the RCN, it's the first time in their 106-year history that they've balloted members for industrial action because of the pay rise offered – *less* than the five per cent above inflation they say we should get. Welcome to power, Rishi Sunak. I can't fucking wait.'

My heart dropped, knowing I was not part of the fight.

'That is bad timing . . .' I said.

'Perfect timing, I'd say. The management can't throw us under the bus when they have a crisis to deal with.'

'Well, they threw me under the bus,' I snorted. 'I lost my job. I can't even begin to tell you the chain reaction it's had.'

Mercedes looked down. She grabbed the kettle, freshly boiled, and placed it on the counter. She dropped two teabags into mugs, then expertly poured in water. All this talk of the RCN was not something I could process.

'They shouldn't have named you,' she whispered, staring into the distance. 'That was wrong. That bloody *Gazette* and Farah, she loves stirring things up.'

Mercedes spooned sugar into the teas, metal clinking against clay.

'Do you know Farah?' I asked.

Mercedes shook her head. 'Only through you.' Mercedes turned, replacing the kettle. I noticed how she avoided my eye. 'Is that a bottle of gin in the corner?' She giggled, wiping a drop of spilt tea from the counter. 'You are a sneaky one, you know that?'

She walked over, handing me a mug.

'Thanks,' I said.

I stared into my tea: strong, just how I liked it, and right now, very much needed.

'Thought you might enjoy this: Preeti got into a spat with security for leaving the ward door open. Can you imagine? Any psychopath could've walked in.'

'Surprising,' I said, picturing the ward, the beds, the front desk . . . Dev and Leroy. 'Preeti is usually so careful.'

'Yeah, but she's tired. We all are. She's struggling to think straight.' Mercedes stared down into her mug. 'Of course, Sandra is stomping around like she's in charge. Even about the strikes. I'm not saying she's wrong to want to get things organised. But I don't remember anyone appointing *her* in charge of the rest of us. Plus, you'd never believe what else . . .'

'What else?' I took another sip.

'Jimmi – nearly lost it with Ravi.'

I sat straighter. '*Ravi?*'

*Ravi who dobbed me in. Ravi, that bastard.*

'In the canteen.' Mercedes took a gulp of tea. 'Ravi is creepy. I hate the way he crawls around the place, checking supplies like we're stealing,' she said. 'They're being more careful.'

She glanced down.

I felt a rush of overwhelm just then, like everything was hurtling towards me like a train. I felt an urge to tell Mercedes the truth. But there was no way I could do that.

There was a knock on the door.

Mercedes looked up. 'Are you expecting someone?'

'Might be Nikolaus.' I placed my mug on the coffee table, feeling jittery and nervous. It would be around now that Nikolaus would be finishing up, making his way over.

Another knock, this one harder. I hesitated.

Maybe it was the police.

'Aren't you going to answer it?' Mercedes sounded a bit annoyed, since she'd made the effort to see me, assuming this time was exclusive. All I kept thinking was that the police were here. They'd finally caught up with me. They wanted me arrested. Maybe they'd traced the call to emergency services. But how could they? I'd used Leroy's phone.

'Nina. It is me!'

It was Nikolaus.

Mercedes peered at me as I walked towards the door, unlocking the latch, feigning casual.

Nikolaus burst in, agitated, short of breath. 'I am

waiting outside for a long time. It is not a good idea to keep me waiting in our situation. I have finished work – and I come here urgently.' He grabbed me and kissed me hard. I stood dumbfounded. He entered the living area but stopped abruptly when he caught sight of Mercedes.

Nikolaus turned to me, then to Mercedes, a hand running through his hair. 'I'm sorry . . . I did not know you have a visitor.'

'Don't mind me.' Mercedes sniggered.

I flinched, slipping past Nikolaus. 'Nikolaus and I . . . we're making some arrangements for us to do a few things over the next few days,' I said.

Mercedes beamed.

I took his jacket as he peeled it off, hanging it up on the wall beside the shoe stand. I moved to a spare chair in the corner. Nikolaus stood there, his hands wedged firmly in his pockets, his shoulders stiff, waiting for her to leave, with, presumably, thoughts of how he'd manage the inconvenience if she didn't.

'Maybe we go away for a few days,' he said, turning to me.

Mercedes glanced down. 'How nice.'

I thought I'd detected a slight tone of condemnation from my friend just then. I couldn't work out if Mercedes was secretly happy for me or just being overprotective.

'How long have you two been dating?' she said.

'Nearly three weeks,' said Nikolaus.

I observed how she raised her eyebrows. 'And already you're going away? Must be love.'

That was definitely sarcasm.

'It's early days,' I interjected, moving to the sofa, taking a seat. Nikolaus walked over to join me.

'Like I said, that night at the pub. You had to leave because, well, you always leave. We met, coincidentally, and we just sort of . . . hit it off.' I smiled at Mercedes. Two could play this game. 'We've been seeing each other, on and off, ever since. It's going well – isn't that right, Nikolaus?'

Nikolaus nodded.

'We are spending some time together,' he said. He moved closer, placing his arm around me. 'Not *on and off.* It is very serious.'

Mercedes cleared her throat. 'Right, well . . . that's lovely for you both.'

I looked down. So, this is how it would be. Two women moving on, departing from a childhood friendship.

I moved to the kitchen sink, pouring the rest of my tea down the drain. I tried not to think about Mercedes' startled reaction as she grabbed her handbag.

Nikolaus made himself comfortable, switching on the TV – anything for a bit of noise and I welcomed it.

'Maybe, if you don't mind, you leave Nina and me to talk in private?' he said casually. 'We must discuss some important matters.' He didn't look up; he was fixed to the screen. He didn't see that Mercedes was preparing to leave anyway.

'Oh?' Mercedes said. 'I didn't realise you'd moved in here as well. Be careful, Nina. He's assuming a bit too much, don't you think? He'll have you running his errands next.'

'He didn't mean it like that, did you, Nikolaus?' I heard how my voice trembled. 'We do need to talk, though. It *is* a bit personal. We can catch up later, can't we?' My eyes pleaded for Mercedes to understand.

Mercedes froze, then smiled. 'I get it. I don't want to get in the way of you two lovebirds. I must get on, anyhow.'

I walked her to the front door, where she grabbed my arm and pulled me outside.

We stood there, each waiting for the other to speak. The landing was cold, the floor burning the soles of my feet.

'What was that?' she whispered.

'What was what?'

'*That?*'

'A man I like,' I said.

'You don't say.' Mercedes slapped her forehead. 'It's all moving a bit fast, isn't it? Are you sure you know what you're doing?'

'Sure, I do. I really like him.'

Mercedes looked down, rubbing her chin. 'Don't get me wrong, Nina. I am happy for you. It's just that he feels a bit . . . *intense*. I'm not sure of the timing of this relationship after everything going on at Newgate. He puts me on edge, if I'm being completely honest.'

'He works in the mortuary,' I said, 'it's to be expected. Nikolaus is just a bit different, that's all. It's the reason I like him. Besides, he's like me. Grew up without a family – was abandoned. He gets it. We're the same.'

'I get it. But I hope you scrub yourself afterwards. Burn a bit of sage. Open the window to let the ghosts escape.' Mercedes stared at me deadly serious, then chuckled, slapping my arm.

'That's not funny,' I spat.

'It's a joke! Look, I get that there's a connection. And that you've not been yourself recently, after everything with Dev and those stupid, malicious investigations. But just be careful, okay?'

If only Mercedes knew the half of it, I thought.

'He's been helpful and useful when I needed him around.'

'That right?'

'Yeah.'

'What did he do, put up a few shelves, move the furniture about? No one really knows much about him – or his life before Levinstone. He says he's from Germany, but can you be sure?'

I felt my face burn. 'The accent is a dead giveaway. And, just so I'm clear, do you think sleeping with a married woman for handouts is better?'

Mercedes flinched.

I glanced down. 'Sorry. I didn't mean that.'

Mercedes clenched her jaw. 'I haven't got time for this, alright? I've got to go.'

She stomped down the stairs, calling after her. 'I've always been here for you,' she said. 'Just remember that. We still need to look out for one another, even though we're adults.'

I stared down at my crooked feet, then turned to push the front door open.

The warmth of my flat was comforting.

'She is gone?' Nikolaus stood up expectantly as I entered. 'We need to finalise the arrangement with Leroy,' he said.

I collapsed back onto the sofa with him. 'I also need to return to the park to make sure I've got his phone and the knife I . . .' It was all too much.

I placed my phone down on the table.

'Stefan will help us,' he said.

'You told him?'

'Yes. I see him earlier.'

I shot up. 'What did you say, exactly?'

'Only that there is a body, and he must burn it but that he must not ask any questions. For his own protection.'

I got up, leaning over Nikolaus, and grabbed his arm. 'Nik, are you *absolutely* sure we can trust him?'

'Nina. We already discuss this. There is no other option.'

I shook my head. 'I don't know about this . . .'

'We can trust him. You must trust *me*.'

I felt my throat constrict.

'He will burn the body. No one will ever know. I already spoke with him. He will do it.'

The more I thought about it, the more it made sense.

'It will be like a funeral to show . . . respect.'

I nodded. 'You're right. Burning is the best option because it will remove evidence.' I swallowed hard, my eyes darting around the room.

'No body, no crime. Only missing persons.' He stood, placing an arm around my shoulder. 'We do this together. We are a team, now.'

I thought of Mercedes, how she'd been a sister to me. But now Nikolaus was here. Life was changing.

Just then, my phone pinged. I pulled it from my back pocket. Glancing down, I noticed a text from an unknown number:

+447757108376

*Hello. My name is Sid Waqar from Waqar Hassall. I'm acting as legal counsel for Mrs Manisha Shah in connection with the death of her son, Dev Shah. I hope you don't mind me texting you, but I thought this more convenient. I wondered if you could call me. We'd like to speak to you.*

I wondered how Sid had got my number.

'There is a problem?' Nikolaus searched my face.

'No problem,' I said, replacing my phone in my pocket. 'It's just Mercedes.'

He stared at me, confused. This was not the right time to talk to Nikolaus about Newgate. We already had one problem to deal with. The last thing I needed was another complication.

'This plan is perfect,' I said, sitting back down. '*Missing persons* is difficult to solve and to prosecute. It will be easier for you, for us. So . . . let's do it.'

He smiled, settling next to me.

'Thank you, Nikolaus.'

For a second, my body trembled, blown by how confident and expert he now appeared. I knew he was only trying to help, that I had done this to him. But I couldn't help thinking: did Mercedes have a point? Did I really know everything there was to know about him?'

'You haven't done this before, have you?' I asked after a while.

He snorted.

'Promise?'

'I am helping you, Nina,' he said. 'I do this for us, for our future. We are the same, you and me. We have the same destiny, I think. We meet for a reason.'

He was calm, unflinching, as if he'd had a conversation with God and had reached an important conclusion.

'When are we doing this?' It needed to happen fast. I couldn't leave Leroy in my car like that.

'Later tonight, very late, we move Leroy to the crematorium. From there, Stefan will take over. For him, this is normal.'

He took hold of my arm, and I realised how much I needed Nikolaus now, how good and natural it felt. I needed to stop doubting myself. I needed to move on – to trust him. He'd done so much already to protect me.

'You are not alone in this,' he said, 'please don't forget it.'

To hear him say that meant everything to me. I'd waited a lifetime to be brave enough to let someone in fully.

I jumped up, my next thought about cleaning the car, and how satisfying that would be. I'd use a new cloth, a tub of bleach, plastic gloves, a thick sponge with a scouring pad.

'I'll clean the car after we . . .'

Nikolaus nodded. 'Yes, it would be sensible.'

'We will need to go to the park first, the crematorium afterwards.' I looked up at Nikolaus. 'We can't make any mistakes.'

We showered and changed, and after a coffee and a short nap, I drove us to the park. The roads were clear but wet. I tapped a finger nervously on the steering wheel as I turned into the park entrance.

Nikolaus shuffled in his seat; he said he didn't feel like talking.

'I won't be long,' I said.

He nodded.

I pulled up into a parking bay and ran out of the car, the cold hitting me in the face, the late hours of the evening crisp and biting. As I approached the bin, a slow panic unravelled. I saw a flash of that night, the shooting, Leroy staggering. In a split second, my life had changed.

I switched on the torch on my phone and shone it inside the plastic-lined basin. It was empty but for an old McDonald's paper bag. I desperately rummaged inside, my hand wet and cold, brushing against the plastic lining . . . nothing.

I looked up to my left and saw a sign on the wall. 'Park Rubbish Collection: Monday, Thursday, Sunday 2 p.m.'

# 29

The knife and phone were gone. There was nothing we could do about that. If we executed the next phase well, there would at least be no reason for the police to go looking for them.

By now it was 2 a.m. and that drive to the crematorium was the longest I'd ever known. The vehicle weighed down at the back made everything feel slower.

Nikolaus had taken over the wheel. My hands trembled. I felt him glance at me often during the drive along the main road, the wheel steady in his hands. The early morning, dark and solemn.

I glanced out of the window. This town, the one I loved so much, now seemed tired and distant. I felt detached; the soul of it had been ripped out. A wash of liquid light splayed yellow against the concrete pavements. The streets were eerily empty. Fried chicken shops, jerk joint huts, the Roti Maker restaurant, largely missing its people. There were a few stragglers out on the streets – possibly selling drugs or doing other dodgy deals – frequenting the darkest places.

I thought of Leroy, his barbed-wire tattoo, that look in his eyes when I plunged the knife in. It was as if, all along, he'd seen who I was. What I was capable of doing.

The car slowed before a red traffic light.

Nikolaus stared out front, observing a moth dancing under a street light. An old grubby suitcase was left torn and soaking by the bin.

'There's still time to go to the police,' Nikolaus said. 'If you change your mind.'

'Have you changed your mind?'

'No.'

'Neither have I.'

'Good. I was just checking.'

He sighed, fumbling around his jacket pocket for his cigarettes as the engine vibrated. I watched the smoke rise and curl around his head like streaky fingers.

'Do you mind opening the window?' I said, suddenly irritated by the fact that he'd assumed it was okay to smoke in my car without my permission.

He glared at me, as if to say *Really? After what we just did?*

'I can't breathe, Nikolaus. Please. I don't want to snap. Just do it.'

He gripped the steering wheel; the light turned amber, green. He wound down the window, flicking his cigarette onto the pavement, and pressed down on the gas.

'You must stay calm, Nina. We must be focused.'

I scrolled through my phone as he drove, marvelling at how Nikolaus could remain so calm. I reread the message from Sid Waqar to distract myself, deliberating whether I should reply. But it was hardly the right time.

I saved his number. For a moment I allowed myself to ponder whether the investigation led by Manisha would land me in yet more trouble.

Nikolaus stared at the road ahead and continued the drive in silence. The car joined a short line of unexpected traffic. I wound down my window, comforted by the cold night prickling my face. Nikolaus took out his phone.

'You can't use your phone while driving,' I said.

He grunted then positioned it near the handbrake. 'I'm simply checking for messages from Stefan.'

I was in no position to question Nikolaus. I was vulnerable, and here he was, someone I cared for deeply, taking excellent care of a delicate situation. I wondered what might have happened had Nikolaus and I never met. But then again, Leroy would still be dead. Nothing about that would change.

I placed my hand on his thigh as he drove, weaving through traffic. 'For a second, I thought you might be recording me.' I laughed nervously.

He raised an eyebrow.

'To use as evidence against me if we get caught,' I said. That voice of self-sabotage, once again.

'Still, you do not trust me, c'mon.'

'Of course I do. We're here, aren't we?'

Leroy was also here, in the back. I wondered whether he was listening to our conversation.

'It bothers me that I don't know anything about Stefan,' I said. There, on the main road, the world somehow felt enormous.

'We are like brothers,' Nikolaus said. 'We went for studies together in Berlin. Then we came to London. For a short time, we lived together.' He glanced at me. 'I told you the story already.'

His story sounded familiar. In some ways, it was reminiscent of my friendship with Mercedes. Fortuitous, perhaps. Yet another confirmation that he and I were alike.

'We are close,' he said, his voice lowered. He swallowed,

clenching his jaw, turning the steering wheel sharply to enter a side road.

The road was flanked by barren oak trees, big, well-to-do detached family houses. At the end of the road stood the crematorium, a Tudor house with a discreet commercial shopfront. A sprawling building that resembled an upmarket GP surgery for middle-class doctors. Double doors, blacked-out windows.

Nikolaus parked under a giant oak tree.

I was breathing harder, faster, the prospect of what was to come now stomach-sickeningly close. 'Are you *sure* there will be no trace of him if we do this? You're absolutely sure?'

Nikolaus nodded. 'Stephan is an expert; his work is clean. He has found a coffin. There will be no after-effect. No ghosts, even.' He chuckled.

I figured it was an attempt to make light of the situation.

'Remember what we agree. He and I will remove the body from the car. You come after ten minutes. We need to take him to the back and put him in the coffin. You do not need to see this. When you come inside the building, wait in the front. Stefan will burn the body. Then it will be completed.' He sighed.

I grabbed Nikolaus's arm. 'I'm so grateful to you for sparing me the finer details. But you know too why I need to watch his body burn. It's so that I *know* it's over. I just want us to move on with our lives.'

'I understand.' He stared into my eyes and smiled. 'I think it is Stefan's preference, also. He feels it would be respectful. He takes his job very seriously.'

I swallowed, my throat scratching. 'Then we're all agreed.'

Nikolaus climbed out of the car.

I sat still and stared out of the window. A figure emerged from the crematorium. Momentarily, he stood in the doorway, tall and thin, wearing a black polo and navy jeans. His oversized trench coat was open, cuffs falling below his wrists. The light in the doorway struck his face. He appeared more French than German with his long pointed nose, dark wavy hair – somehow stereotypically, you could say, he looked more generically European. There was something about him that spoke of his upbringing, too – cultured and refined. I imagined him drinking a glass of red Bordeaux in front of a log fire, discussing art, truffles, economic reform, prosperity for the people. A far cry from a man who buried and burned bodies.

I checked my watch. It was now 2.30 a.m.

My heart was thumping hard in my chest. I rolled my seat back and closed my eyes to settle my breath. When I opened them again, Stefan was at the back of the car. The two men greeted one another, Nikolaus patting Stefan on the back. Stefan, beaming a smile. He was animated; the kind of man who did most of his talking with his hands.

Nikolaus pointed to the boot, then to the front. Stefan met my eyes and waved, but he did not approach. It felt like, given the circumstances, he thought it best for us to remain at a distance. Stefan said something to Nikolaus and rushed off towards the home's entrance.

After a minute or so, Stefan returned with a trolley. He wheeled it towards the car; Nikolaus ran to assist him. They grabbed either side, manoeuvring it so that it was positioned at the back. Their movements were like wild animals rustling in the woods for food. Amid the rickety sound of wheels, the clanging of metal, I felt increasingly unsettled. I wanted this over and done with as quickly as possible.

I heard mumbled voices, grunting, the same tone I'd heard from Nikolaus when I'd had him close, but these grunts belonged to Stefan, I was quite sure.

'Es ist schwierig. Sein Körper ist steif,' said Nikolaus.

'Leg ihn auf den trolley . . . und wir werden ihn los,' replied Stefan.

It did occur to me, as they pushed the trolley up the path, that I could drive off. Abandon the two men, make this all their problem. But I was kidding myself because there was no way I could leave Nikolaus now. We were in this together; we'd promised.

I waited a few minutes, like we'd agreed, and then got out of the car.

I walked towards the Tudor house, entering the hall, decorated with swirly velvet wallpaper, a leather chesterfield suite: two armchairs, a sagging four-seater. The air smelled of dry wood, and strangely, of cinnamon.

I took a few steps. At the end of the hall, I turned left, entering a quiet room lit up in scarlet. A lone candle flickered on a side table next to a depressing vase of dried flowers. Here, the air smelled of ash and sage and old ladies' linen. If I was not mistaken, something like rosemary also faintly lingered. A window was open; grey curtains billowed in a light breeze. I moved to the front row and sat down on a velvet chair, attempting to make myself comfortable.

This room was styled like a chapel, just like the one in Newgate Hospital where they'd removed all the religious symbols to make it feel spiritually universal. But here, I felt terribly alone. No sermon, no parable, no prayer to be recited on behalf of others. I was a nurse, here and everywhere; that's all I ever wanted to be. But I had done the unthinkable, killing a man, when I ought to have saved him.

I heard voices in the back. Fifteen minutes had passed. The moon was discernible through the trees, the milky white sketching silver shadows onto the grey curtains.

There were rummaging sounds, and then in front, I saw grey curtains part. Before me lay an empty stage, strangely symbolic of life drawing to an end.

Stefan ambled in. Up close, not so attractive. He was shabby and worn, nervously chewing on gum.

Nikolaus entered the room just behind him and shuffled close. He took a seat next to me, lowering his head.

'I do not like funerals,' he said, his voice faint and sullen.

Stefan turned his back, typing onto a digital pad on the wall. He paused before pressing a flashing green button. A beep sounded; a rumble began. It was like the sound you heard in an airport from a baggage claim conveyor belt.

Before long, a shiny, black coffin came rolling out. Flickers of candlelight reflected against the mirror polish.

During those long sixty seconds of silence, I uttered, for the first time in my life, a silent prayer. I prayed Leroy would pass safely to the other side. That he would come to understand that what had happened was inevitable.

Stefan made a sign of the cross, touching, sequentially, his forehead, lower chest, the balls of both shoulders. Nikolaus clenched his eyes closed, but I continued to watch the coffin disappear. In my mind, I heard the spit and crackle of burning wood, as the metal doors to the crematorium closed.

# 30

I climbed the stairs to my flat, fumbling for my keys. I intended to fall asleep for a very long time to avoid returning to reality. I had no job, no income, and soon it would be Christmas. For a second, I figured that maybe I should find work in retail like Sunil. But overcome with tiredness as I was, I knew I didn't have it in me.

Inside, I kept the flat dark, spending the following nights staring out onto the empty street below. I ignored my messages, even the ones from Nikolaus. The familiarity of my surroundings offered no comfort nor reprieve from the shock of it all.

After four days, I sat down at the end of my bed, reading the latest text Mercedes had sent me earlier that afternoon. She wanted to know when we could meet up.

*Not being funny, but you've been acting strange since you've been going out with Nikolaus! We're friends, and friends come first, remember? What is going on?? Why so silent?? xxx*

The phone was warm in my hand, and in that moment, I was compelled to dial a number. I knew well, it was the only call I could make, on the off chance that it might save me from myself.

It rang several times before someone answered.

'Hello?'

The woman's voice was deep and hoarse. In the background, murmuring street sounds, traffic, the angry roar of a bus.

'Who is this?' she said.

A shiver ran through me.

'Why are you calling this number so late?'

That voice, that tone. There was no way it could be her. It was too cruel, detached, somewhat cockney. A Londoner, for sure. But she sounded like someone from a rougher part of town. One of those voices you'd hear at the end of a drunken night.

Silent and numb, I was unable to speak.

'Are you going to say anything? For fuck's sake!'

'Mum . . .?'

The words were caught in my throat.

The woman sighed. 'Listen, I need to make a call, and you've got the wrong number, alright? You're calling a telephone box.'

With that, she hung up.

And so, I did the only thing I could to keep my mind occupied and to maintain some semblance of normality and sanity, some control over an otherwise precarious situation. I scrubbed my flat clean, more deeply than I'd ever managed before. Crawling on my hands and knees, I scrubbed every inch, corner and crack, with a sponge and toothbrush. When I was done, I dusted shelves. I then made my way to the car, braving the cold, carrying a bucket of boiling water, cloths and cleaning products. Scrubbing the dashboard, polishing the windows, I soaped the carpets and mopped up leftover dried blood. I removed the seat covers to boil-wash them with strong detergent.

Afterwards, with a sense of serenity and satisfaction, and seated alone in the dark, only the flicker of the TV and the hum of the washing machine turning in the background, I attempted to sleep. When that failed, I tried to force myself into a slumber by drinking. Gin, brandy, the odd bottle of cheap wine. Anything to stop the flashbacks.

The following day, when I pulled out my phone, nursing the worst hangover known to man, I saw I'd received a text message:

> Sid Waqar
> *Hello. This is Sid Waqar again from Waqar Hassall. I'm acting as legal counsel for Mrs Manisha Shah in connection with the death of her son, Dev Shah. I don't know if you got my earlier text. I would really appreciate it if you could call me. I need to speak to you.*

I dialled his number and made an appointment. His office was not far from Newgate Hospital, he said. I took the bus, wanting to avoid that stench of death in the car which, despite my cleaning, was still very much present.

Sid's office was located on Russell Street, in a brown shoebox building, windows too small to offer any decent lighting. I walked through the main entrance in a clean tracksuit approaching the siren-red doors. My jacket was heavy and wet from rain. The uniformed security guard remained indifferent to my arrival, directing me to the lift with a grunt of irritation.

The waiting area in reception was pristine white. Hung on the wall was a giant poster of three African women in glorious yellow costumes, tending to a child. 'It takes a village', read the caption.

I gave my name at the front desk to a woman more interested in reading her horoscopes than receiving me. I took a seat on the blue sofa and crossed my legs. Leaning forward, I riffled through a fan of leaflets.

*Justice for all*, one read.

I picked it up:

*We are a unique firm for locals who have been injured, discriminated against, or had their human rights violated. We are also national and international, specialising in personal injury, human rights, clinical negligence, employment, and group claims.*

'Nina Dabral?'

Hearing my name called made me jump.

A man wearing a shiny grey wedding suit appeared and reached out his hand. I replaced the leaflet as the man tipped his head, pursing his lips like he perfectly understood the blank expression on my face.

He directed me into a side office where the shelves ran floor to ceiling, stocked with files, leather-bound books, a few awards and trophies. A giant conference table stood in the middle of the room. To my left, a large window. I moved closer and saw it overlooked the entrance to an African jeweller.

A woman entered the room wearing a black salwar kameez. She asked me whether I'd like something to drink, and I thanked her, requesting a black coffee. She nodded and laughed at my insistence she spoon in at least three sugars.

The door closed and Sid and I stared at one another. He cleared his throat, and we sat down. I folded my arms, feeling suddenly defensive.

'You're probably wondering what this is all about.'

'You could say that.' I tried to make myself comfortable, rearranging myself in my seat, attempting to appear relaxed in this strangely stiff environment.

'Like I mentioned in my text, we're representing Manisha Shah in connection with her son, Dev Shah, a former patient of yours.'

'Got nothing more to say. I've been fired.'

He pulled a notepad towards him, carefully removing a pen from his pocket. Something about the way he held it, pointing the nib in my direction, reminded me of Farah. 'That's just it, see . . .' He smiled knowingly. 'An independent investigation was carried out by us into Dev's death. The outcome contradicts the findings confirmed by the hospital in their mandatory investigation.'

'I'm sorry?'

He paused as if by instinct, knowing I'd need a moment to digest this new piece of information.

'I don't understand,' I said.

'Let's just say the evidence you gathered was most revealing.'

I froze. 'What evidence? I don't know anything about any evidence. Don't go throwing around accusations.'

'It's okay,' said Sid. 'You're safe here. But could you, for the record, confirm what you believe happened?'

'No, I will not!' I spat. My defences rose higher. 'I've already gone through it once. As far as I'm concerned, it's over. I can't begin to tell you how much this has fucked up my life. I don't work at Newgate. They fired me, like I said. I want to move on with my life.'

Sid leaned back in his chair, his face contorting. A vein under his eyebrow throbbed; his left eye flickered.

I was about to get up to leave, but he urged me to remain seated.

'I understand how upset you are.'

'You've no idea.'

'I have some idea. Look, I'll get straight to it. Dev died of sepsis.'

I was stunned. The breath in my chest fluttered like a trapped bird.

'That is strictly off record. Our investigation focused on how it was missed, where responsibility lies for it.'

'That doesn't make sense. Bloods were carried out . . . They found *nothing*. Sudden cardiac death. That's what they said in the meeting.' My mind raced; my eyes crawled over the deep pile in the brown carpet.

'SCD is an outcome rather than a cause. That's the discrepancy and key error in the report.'

'You mean the coroner's report was wrong?'

'The coroner focused on the immediate cause of death, as they often do. Technically, he was right to report cardiac arrest. Underlying sepsis was not highlighted in any of Dev's medical records – his bloods or CT scan – and he had no reason to question it. But our investigation revealed that severe sepsis and septic shock was the *cause* of SCD.

Cardiac arrest was a late-stage complication.'

My eyes darted about the room.

'The next question we asked ourselves was, why did Dev's records not show sepsis? That's where your efforts were helpful.'

I searched his face. 'You're not making any sense. None of the blood tests confirmed sepsis, nor the CT scan. Why would there be doubt about that when we have those results and the coroner didn't question it?'

Sid licked his lips. 'Let's deal with the bloods. See, there can only be three explanations as to why sepsis was not detected earlier. One: blood tests were not carried out, as assumed, by MediCentral, which would be nonsensical because we know they were – and we know there were results reported. Two: bloods *were* carried out but the results were wrong. This raises questions of why and how. Three: tests were carried out and were right, but results were deliberately falsified by the time they were logged on Dev's record, at Newgate.'

'What?'

'Given what had been uncovered, a new supplier forced through by the CEO – already unethical, with new processes implemented. We knew there was bound to be something that stinks.' He looked at me knowingly. 'So, we followed the dirty trail and found exactly where it happened. Short story, had those test results – the correct results – reached you and the doctors, sepsis would have been detected. Dev may have lived.'

I was speechless. 'But I *personally* did those tests. I took bloods myself. I inserted the needle into Dev's vein, labelled the bottles and sent them down the chute into the lab. The whole process was a chore – and certainly some of the results took their sweet time coming back – but I followed the process correctly and tried to make it work.'

'But most of the testing was done off-site by MediCentral. Only the urgent bloods needing a one-hour turnaround were carried out on site.'

'Of course I know that. What are you suggesting, exactly?'

Sid rearranged himself as if building to a final reveal. 'The results arrived at the lab, and were double-checked by staff before being logged onto a patient's record.'

I saw a flash of Dev's face in the mortuary. Patches of blue on his skin.

'The MediCentral roll-out was controversial for all manner of reasons. But the main one was that no one wanted it. People feared losing their jobs. Lab staff feared that the most. So of course, we dug there, at what went wrong. How it was that *we* found sepsis in Dev's post-mortem, but that sepsis didn't show up in the bloods. Now, the MediCentral records on Dev's samples did show sepsis. Those were correct. But when the results were logged at Newgate, the results showed all-clear. That made it obvious that the results were interfered with.' Sid shook his head. 'Transpires, two members of staff in the lab altered the test results. Liam Jackson and Arvin Patel. They wanted the roll-out to fail. They feared the roll-out more than anyone.'

*Arvin . . . Liam.*

Sid sat back in his chair and sighed. 'It's a terrible situation, Nina. One that demands justice for poor Dev, and for you too, caught up in it.'

I could hardly believe what I was hearing. I recalled Dev's

mottled skin – that's what it was. Sepsis!

'It's a difficult economic climate,' said Sid. 'They took matters into their own hands, sabotaged the implementation of outsourcing bloods so that MediCentral appeared incompetent.'

I heard a faint ringing in my ears as I recalled my conversation with Arvin and Liam:

*Today, routine and gold standard; tomorrow, all blood testing. Next time you see us, we might not have jobs.*

'We know Manisha approached you a bit hostile . . .'

'Not a bit, a *lot*,' I snapped.

'I can tell you she deeply regrets doing that. Your efforts revealed that Richard was profiting from MediCentral's implementation,' continued Sid, 'that he received further financial incentives for increasing testing numbers. It's sickening to think about it, and tragic that despite a higher number of tests, none of them saved Dev. The implementation of MediCentral caused corruption at staff level.'

'But that still doesn't explain the CT scan Dev had. Why didn't sepsis show in that?'

Sid licked his lips. 'A CT scan can be equivocal or can be misinterpreted, as you know. In Dev's case, it was carried out without radio-opaque dye, which unfortunately made the scan less thorough than if dye had been used. Manisha did not want Dev to ingest contrast solution. If you recall, she point-blank refused it.'

'God.' I remembered that night.

'It was a perfect storm of issues. All of it resulting in the loss of a young man's life.'

We sat silent for a while as the air around us swelled.

'How did the information I sent to Farah reach you?' I said, quietly – almost a whisper. 'That is a huge violation. I trusted her.'

'Nina, if she hadn't shared it, Dev would not receive justice – and there would have been more deaths. We don't need to know how you got hold of it, but rest assured, you are protected. We won't expose you. Here, have some water.'

Sid poured me a glass from a jug on the table. I moved towards him and sat down, still unsure whether I could trust him.

'They blamed me . . .' I said, the anger rising. 'I was made a scapegoat when they had no right.'

I lowered my head. *I knew it. I knew something was off.*

'You're not without blame.' Sid paused. 'We know about the morphine, the other professional complaints made against you. But that doesn't mean you were responsible for Dev's death. That's an important distinction. You tried your best. You gathered the information that helped expose Richard. The situation is bigger and more complex. You got caught up in it. It's important you hold on to that.'

I wanted to cry, but I fought back the tears.

'You might want some legal advice,' said Sid quietly, matter of fact. 'We'd be happy to offer it to you, pro bono. The number of cases brought against the NHS is enough to keep us busy and well funded for many years.'

I stared down at my hands, resting in my lap.

'They fired me,' I said. 'That doesn't change, does it?'

He smiled. 'You might receive a formal letter from the hospital offering to throw you a line. With the sheer magnitude of corruption at Newgate, the PR damage is a nightmare for them. They'll want to be seen offering better support to those nurses caught up in the fallout of the Medi-Central roll-out.' He grunted. 'No one would blame you if you didn't want to indulge them. Richard has brought shame on the hospital. But there were shortfalls in duties of care for which you *are* responsible. So this might be, overall, a good outcome for you.'

He stood up and I stood up too.

'You could get your job back. If they don't offer it to you, we could take them on, force their hand. You can still be a nurse. From what I hear, you're otherwise very good.'

I felt faint and unsteady on my feet. I was being given a second chance after everything I did.

'We're here if you want to talk again about anything.' Sid walked me to the door. 'If you see Farah, do give her my regards. She's a brilliant journalist. Been instrumental in exposing Newgate. She's going to have a field day with all of this.'

For a second, I couldn't help but admire Farah, the connections she'd built all over town. She was everywhere: in the streets, the wards, the lawyer's office. But she'd exposed me without my consent. She was not to be trusted.

Sid led me out of the office and to the lift. On the ground floor, I made my way out of the building feeling sick. I kept seeing Maria stomping around Florence Nightingale, paying close attention to patients admitted, tests being carried out. Unknowingly complicit in the corruption too, just like we all were.

Outside, I walked to the car park in a daze. I remembered the coffee I'd requested, which hadn't appeared. I dialled Farah's number. She answered after only one ring and got straight to it.

'I'm glad you called, Nina. I've been wanting to speak to you.' Her voice was calm, assured: a woman who had gotten what she'd wanted all along.

'Presumably you've spoken to Sid?' she asked.

'I've just seen him and—'

'The truth always gets out,' she said. 'I couldn't use the evidence you'd sent for the article because, well . . . you know how personal relationships cloud decisions. But this is better. I hope you understand why it was important to pass it on. You can trust Sid. I promise.'

I scanned the car park, two cars in two bays.

'This story . . . is *huge*,' she said. 'Believe me when I say I will be going big with it – and for sure, with another paper. My editor can go jump in the river.'

The rest of the car park was empty, the concrete littered with cigarette ends. 'Where does that leave me?' I asked. 'I'm still out of a job. My life is a mess. You wrote about me in your sodding paper, and that's what people will remember.'

'Tomorrow, you'll be yesterday's news, or maybe you'll be in the papers for different reasons.' She chuckled. 'I'll make sure I get you a bigger splash – in a more upmarket paper.'

I sat down on a low brick wall.

'You should know – Sid is my cousin,' she said, her tone lowered. 'That's why you can trust him. I wanted him to talk to you. After everything you did, giving me that information, I feel *terrible* that you were named. But at least now you'll be exonerated. *This* is the story I've wanted on Newgate, a story of corruption at the top, of how it trickles down. How otherwise good people get caught up in it, turned, pushed, spat out in a system already strained. Perhaps good and bad aren't what we think in those conditions. We need a nuanced debate.'

I hung up and walked to the other side of the car park, overlooking the green. A group of young boys were tackling each other for a football. I thought of Leroy. Even if I were to be cleared, I could not conceive how life could ever return to what it was.

I sent Nikolaus a text, telling him I desperately missed him. We'd had enough time apart, but now, I needed him back.

I had murdered a man. No amount of a story, retold, would change that. I killed him because of what I thought he did. I was hardly innocent. But now I saw how wrong I'd been about Dev's death, its connection to Leroy. Perhaps even to Balraj. I had blamed the wrong man.

# 31

'It is good, yes? Maybe you get your job back, and we continue to live as normal.'

We were standing in my flat. Nickolaus held me close. His face was filmed with a shine having rushed to see me from work. I could smell Newgate Hospital baked into the pores of his leather jacket, that stale scent of empty days.

'They haven't written to me or called me in yet,' I said. 'I can't believe what Sid told me about Arvin and Liam. How Richard's greed and corruption infected everyone.'

Nikolaus pulled me closer. 'It is very terrible what he did. He was supposed to be our leader. A letter will come, I'm sure. They will not want to make it look worse.'

I sighed, closing my eyes. 'Maybe now the right story will be told,' I said. 'Maybe I won't look so bad.' I felt self-righteous, reflecting on how I'd been portrayed, how wrong and unfair it was, until, of course, I remembered what I'd done to Leroy.

Our fingers knotted; a trace of fresh lemon disinfectant scent unfurled.

'Promise me you will not leave me again,' Nikolaus said. I felt his breath brush my ear. 'I cannot live without you now.'

I closed my eyes, burying my face deep into his chest. I wanted to curl up like a cat at the base of his trunk, to hide under the sprouting branches of his arteries. I yearned to take refuge in the warmth of his beating heart. After everything we'd done, he was the only place I called home. With him, I felt safe from the outside world. 'I promise,' I said.

He kissed my forehead. 'It will be better. I know this in my heart, Nina.'

I pulled away from him, inhaling a chestful of air. I moved to the kitchen counter feeling light-headed, the room rushing around me. I stared into the sink, into the mouth of the dirty drain. A part of me wanted to slip into it, never to emerge from it again.

Nikolaus sighed. 'You are worried what will happen, I know, but it is over.' He slipped behind me, wrapping his arms around my waist. 'We can continue with our lives. Move forward as a couple. Leroy was a bad person.'

But I couldn't move. He must have sensed something was wrong because he tightened his grip.

'Come,' he said.

He painted a stroke down my arm with his fingers, then held my hand, leading me towards the sofa.

He eased me onto the cushion and shuffled close. Drawing his mouth to my lips, I felt the liquid fire of desire wash over us. But after a second, coming back up for air, I pushed him off me.

'Something is wrong?' His face fell.

'I can't,' I said. 'It feels . . .'

'What?'

'It feels wrong, after everything we did. Please don't misunderstand. I'm grateful you were there when I needed you. But this is not normal.'

'Normal?'

'*This.*' I threw an arm into the air. 'Come on, Nikolaus.

How can you act as if nothing's happened? After everything we've been through. How can we have a normal relationship?'

He searched my face for some explanation of what I meant.

'Do you understand?' By now, I was exasperated.

'What kind of foundation is that to build a future on?' I could not understand how Nikolaus could be so . . . *nonchalant.*

'But we are the same, you and me.' His voice plunged into his stomach.

'I need a fresh start. I need to get out. I can't stop thinking about what we did that night. I can't stop seeing . . . blood.'

He swallowed hard, hungrily, thirstily, for me. Then leaned closer. When I failed to respond, to give him anything back, he pulled away and began talking in a dry, measured tone.

'I help you, Nina. I help you when you need me. Not many men would do this for a woman they do not know so well. But I do it because . . . I *feel* something.'

I stood up, moving to the window. *This is it,* I thought. I needed to set him straight. Lay out the ground rules of our relationship and how things would progress from here.

'I'm grateful for what you did. But what I did was wrong. And made so much worse because Leroy was working with the police. I shouldn't have involved you.'

I glanced out of the window at a spider's web hanging in the corner. I considered the intricate threads of my own life. How I'd be spending the rest of my life running away from the murder I'd committed.

Did I even know who Leroy really was? I'd seen him dying. Consumed by anger, I'd killed him mercilessly. And although it's likely he would have died anyway, that did not make it acceptable. Somehow, exposing the corruption of others further exposed me. I was a cold-blooded murderer. It would not be difficult to convince a judge or jury – or even Grace – that I deserved to go to prison.

And yet, knowing I could not change this did not necessarily mean I wanted to hand myself in. Nikolaus was here. He offered the promise of a new life. We'd already disposed of Leroy. Without his body, the police had limited powers. I deserved not to let this one mistake ruin my whole life. I deserved so much better.

Nikolaus stood, pacing the room. He opened his mouth to speak but then closed it again.

'All I'm saying is that I know you helped me. You didn't have to. But just because you did, it doesn't mean you can emotionally blackmail me with it.'

Nikolaus ran a hand through his hair. All I could do was screw my eyes closed. I couldn't bear to witness the car crash that was now my life. Everything was so jumbled.

'When I was younger, all I wanted to lead was a simple life,' I said. I dropped my head into my hands. 'I thought after everything I went through, I could turn it around.'

'But I help you because I love you.' Nikolaus moved closer and held my hand. 'You find yourself in the wrong place, maybe. Me too. I took your phone call, and I came. I involve Stefan. Now we are all mixed in this together.' He squeezed my hand tighter. We stared into one another's eyes. 'I do not regret it,' he said. 'I want to be with you. I mean this.'

My eyes welled. 'I so want it to work, but how can it now?' I searched his eyes, his lips, his face.

'Nobody will know what happened. I will never tell anyone, I promise. We must give ourselves a chance to be happy. We must see what happens.'

I pulled away, shaking my head, and sat down at the kitchen table, my back pressing into my seat. Nikolaus followed, taking a seat opposite me. He grabbed my hand more tightly, unwilling to let it go.

'I will keep our secret for as long as we are together. Not because you force me. Because I want to, Nina.'

I snatched my hand away, even though I wanted him more than ever. 'You're not listening to me. You can't do this; I won't allow it.'

'I love you, Nina.'

I flinched. Hearing those words . . . it meant so much. It was the confirmation I needed. I'd never imagined I might find someone who might love me purely as I was. But here he was, seated in front of me now.

We rose from our chairs, embracing each other awkwardly over the table. Our faces were so close, I felt his breath. I was about to say something but then I heard a knock on the door.

We jolted.

Nikolaus sighed as we straightened.

I made a beeline to the front door to see who it was. As I squinted through the peephole, my body tensed. Mercedes was standing on the doorstep. Her timing could not have been worse.

When I opened the door, she rushed forward.

'I've been so worried about you,' she said, holding me. The familiarity of her sweet strawberry scent, the soft wool from her coat brushed against my face.

She pulled away, holding me at arm's length, then kissed me on the cheek. She entered the flat and I traipsed behind her, staring down at my feet.

Mercedes scoffed when she saw Nikolaus. 'Here again, I see,' she said.

He wedged his hands in his pockets and straightened his back, his face resolute as if preparing a line of defence.

Mercedes turned and winked at me. 'Just can't stay away, can he?'

'We were having lunch,' I said. 'Nikolaus has just finished a shift.'

'You don't say.' Mercedes plopped into a chair at the table as I dragged a beanbag from the corner, dropping it in the centre of the living room.

'A romantic meal for two.' Mercedes smiled mischievously.

'We were . . . discussing some important business.' I plunged into the beanbag, hoping she'd get the hint. The beads rearranged themselves, rustling and patterning as if ready to swallow me.

'*Important business*.' Nikolaus laughed nervously. 'You are so British, Nina.'

'I just meant we were in the middle of chatting about some important stuff,' I replied.

'That right?' Mercedes nodded. 'Discussing funny business, more like.' She giggled.

She was like a child, prodding at our awkwardness. I glanced at Nikolaus's face, his expression visibly aggrieved.

He had just told me he loved me; I did not want to treat him like this.

'So how are you?' I asked Mercedes. Anything to break the tension.

'Oh, you know. The usual. Newgate is still so busy. These past few days in maternity have been manic, what with those babies still needing to be born.'

I watched Nikolaus, feeling a flash of fear as if he might lose it – or say something he shouldn't.

Mercedes poured herself water from the jug, her teeth clinking against the glass as she drank.

'We're all so on edge. Feels like there's been a rise in admissions.'

'I see . . . yeah, of course. At least it's all out in the open,' I mumbled. I was losing my train of thought.

Mercedes placed her glass down, glancing at me strangely. 'Right, you two. What's going on?' Ignoring Nikolaus, she turned to me. 'I want all the details. Spit it out.' She shot Nikolaus a look. 'You must be something. She's not listening properly to a word I've said. She's barely registered I'm here.'

'I do not understand what you are asking,' Nikolaus said shiftily.

Mercedes laughed. 'C'mon, she's utterly besotted with you. You should hear some of her messages: gobbledegook. Or maybe that's gin and not you.'

I glanced down at the carpet, refusing to get entangled in this web, this game of one-upmanship between my two best friends.

'The truth is we're serious about each other,' I said, after a while. I smiled at Nikolaus. 'It's early days, but it feels so right. It feels great.'

Nikolaus smiled back. 'We care for each other very much,' he said.

Mercedes smiled. 'Aw . . . I'm just teasing you both. I'm so happy for you.' She glanced down at her hands. 'I'm just a bit . . . surprised, that's all. Don't take offence, Nik, but you're not her usual type.'

I shot Mercedes a look. 'What the hell does that mean?'

'Nina hasn't gotten serious with anyone until now,' she continued. She stopped when she saw the look on my face. 'Just teasing! But on a serious note, Nikolaus, you had better treat her well or it will be your body I'll be pushing on a trolley down the corridors of Newgate.' She giggled, moving closer to me. I wasn't sure what to make of her mischief and her genuine desire to protect me.

Mercedes removed a strand of hair from my face. 'I just want you to be happy,' she said. 'Whatever that looks like is cool. Just don't forget me, okay? Don't forget who your true friends are.' Mercedes glanced down to the floor. 'I'd better go. I'd seriously hate to get in the way of you both . . .'

She grabbed her bag, and a little dumbfounded, I watched her walk towards the front door.

I got up to see her out, but Mercedes turned as the door opened. 'We need to talk in private,' she whispered. 'I wasn't expecting *he'd* be here . . .'

My shoulders fell. 'Why, what's the matter?'

Mercedes' eyes widened. 'Was it you who exposed the bloody fraud and on-site corruption? There's monumental shit going down. None of us knows the details. You know

Richard's been dismissed? The NHS Counter Fraud Authority has come in, seizing files, carrying out their on-site investigations. They're crawling everywhere, looking into the allegations of his vested interest, the backhanders. Two phlebotomists have been fired, also.'

'I know.'

Mercedes flinched. 'You do? How?'

'It's a long story. Let's just say that Farah has a way of leaking information when it suits her,' I said.

She swallowed. 'None of us knew it was that bad. None of us knows what will happen next.' Mercedes shook her head. 'MediCentral is still in place for now – but how the hell can they continue?' She was thinking. 'Do you think they'll take you back? Have they been in touch?'

'Not yet. But they might. Depends on what happens next,' I said.

Mercedes nodded. 'I still can't believe it . . . I miss you terribly, Nina. Miss seeing you at Newgate. Miss our breakfasts. It's not fair what happened to you when you were just doing your job. It's clear there were bigger problems – and you named it from the start.'

'Thanks,' I said, reaching out my hand, placing it on her shoulder. 'You supported me as I got the information needed.'

Mercedes glanced down. 'You've nothing to be grateful for. I've done nothing – nothing at all. I've not exactly been a good friend, have I? I've been terrible. I'm just sorry . . . for everything.'

I stepped back.

'Sorry? What for? It's not *your* fault I got stitched up by Farah.'

She glanced up, unable to meet my eye. 'It's like you were made the scapegoat for the rest of us . . .'

'Don't think like that.' But in that moment, I thought about what Farah had said. About maternity. The fatalities of mothers and children owing to a lack of adequate care.

'I've got to go,' Mercedes said quickly. 'Call me once lover boy's gone.'

She turned the handle to the door and stepped outside. I watched her leave and closed the door behind her.

In the flat, I pulled out a chair, taking a seat at the table. Nikolaus moved behind me and massaged my shoulders.

'I feel bad lying to Mercedes,' I said. 'She doesn't know the half of it – that things are so much worse.'

Nikolaus poured me a glass of water and handed it to me. I took a few sips, trying hard not to think too much about Leroy.

'She does not need to know,' he said.

'They must be searching for him by now,' I said. 'Given his involvement with the police, they won't let it go. Any minute now, it could all come out . . .'

'He was shot by his own people, yes?' Nikolaus's eyes darted about as if the severity and magnitude of the situation was finally presenting itself.

'We can't be sure. His own people, or enemies. But *snitch* was him snaking on his own, I think.' I moved to the sink and turned on the tap, washing dishes, still thinking about that conversation Leroy had with Barry before he got shot. Staring down, I thought about MediCentral, the blood on my own hands.

Nikolaus approached me from behind, grabbing me by the waist. He pulled me towards him. 'Nina the nurse. Always worrying about things that have not happened.'

There was another knock on the door. I turned off the tap, drying my hot hands on a towel.

'Just me!' It was Mercedes, her voice echoing from the landing outside.

I opened the door.

'I was on the way out, but I saw this—'

She was breathless, waving a brown envelope.

'It says "Newgate" on the front.'

# 32

The corridors of Newgate Hospital were the same as they'd always been. Patients lined up to be seen in A&E. Mothers wandered frantically in the waiting area with sick children. A man in a corduroy suit banged his fists on the reception window as the receptionist kissed her teeth. Her expression said it all: *Go sit down*. Did this man not know? There were at least one hundred other patients waiting before him in the queue with symptoms more serious.

My phone vibrated.

Mercedes 18.50
*So glad you're back! How u feeling??*

Nina 18.51
*A bit strange tbh. Is it my imagination or is A&E worse than it was before I left?*

Mercedes 18.52
*For sure, it's worse after everything. Everyone is so demotivated. But remember, you did nothing wrong! Everyone knows that.*

Walking towards Florence Nightingale ward, with its familiar stale stench of nothingness, its unbearable, suffocating warmth, I found myself taking deep breaths, longing to somehow become one with it. I needed, so desperately, to cling on to what I knew: normality, familiarity, progress. Anything to move forward.

At the entrance, I pressed my card onto the new sensors installed. They'd tightened up security. My card wasn't recognised. I caught sight of Sandra through the glass. She waved at me awkwardly, and I waved back. Then she turned and disappeared around the corner like a ghost.

Barbara approached, smiling, her face earthy and warm. I detected a woman full of empathy and concern. She pressed the green button for me to enter.

'Welcome back,' she said, nudging the door wider to let me in. 'You'll need a new card,' she said. I clutched my card tightly in my hand.

'Thanks,' I said.

'You're okay? Not too nervous?'

I shook my head.

'That's great,' she winked.

Silently, I walked behind her towards her office. Inside, we sat down opposite one another. I grew aware just how shallow my breaths had grown, how my heart stuttered and pounded.

'It was not your fault. I want you to remember that.' Barbara's voice was urgent. 'None of us could have known what was going on here. We all feel cheated and let down by such appalling behaviour.' She winced. 'A man in a position of authority . . . and *bloods* of all things! People I've trusted for years I now question whether I ever really knew in the first place.'

I looked down at my hands. 'You're talking about Liam and Arvin.'

'Richard was supposed to bring in the changes we needed to help us all move forward.' Barbara shook her head. 'The whole hospital needs a reset,' she said. 'We've been set back several years, what with more changes to management. It's going to take at least two years. Maybe three. By then we'll have the results of the public inquiry. It will bring about the greater change we so desperately need. Hopefully, the government will communicate its plan for the NHS by then – if it's still the Tories in power, that is.'

'But what do we do in the meantime?' I asked.

'Well, you're back, which is great. We focus on the present. We carry on as normal. We're committed to giving you the help you need. Least we can do given the circumstances.'

I stared out of the window, struggling to take it all in. So many changes.

'Our job is to help heal the sick. Nothing changes on that front,' she said.

I was outside my body, floating over the woman who no longer felt like she belonged. I could hear Barbara's voice, but it seemed to fade in and out.

'Naturally, given the morphine discrepancies, we are obliged to be cautious. It's to protect you. The counselling, surveillance . . . is all part of the process, too. You understand that, don't you?'

I glanced back at Barbara. 'Sorry?'

'Why you can't have access to the medical supplies room, nor the controlled drugs cabinet. It's just temporary. Just until things settle for you.'

'I understand,' I said, fiddling with my hands, unsure what parts of the conversation I'd missed.

'Excellent.' Barbara shuffled through papers on her desk. 'And remember, there's no judgement. We know how tough it is. Stress does strange things to people. While others are just greedy.'

I scanned the room around me, the walls painted blue. 'Blue?'

'It needed a fresh coat. This is a hospital, Nina. They've no sense of colour!'

We both laughed.

'You're looking well,' Barbara said after a while. 'It wasn't the same here without you. I'm delighted you're back.'

'It's good to *be* back,' I said, and for a second, I meant it, too.

Barbara slapped her hands on her knees, and I jumped.

'Well. I'm just glad we could work this out, that you're okay with a slight change of duties. Remember, if anything feels too much, you can always talk to me about it.' She smiled. 'I think you'll find everyone is hugely supportive.'

I entered the changing room to slip into my scrubs. It felt good to be wearing them again. Moving to the nurse's station, I felt a little more confident. By instinct, I began cleaning the computer keyboard, wiping whatever smear and filth was on those keys, invisible to the human eye, but most definitely smeared on each letter.

*ABCDE.*

I logged into the system with my card and scanned through my to-do list:

Four blood pressure checks, several B12 injections, an ECG, and then some dressings. A patient, Patsy Wood, bed twenty, had been brought in with stitches after a punch-up with another woman in McDonald's over whose meal it allegedly was sitting in the brown paper bag on the counter.

I thought of Farah and glanced at the private room to the side of me. I remembered Leroy's face. That blank expression in his eyes when I saw, up close, he was dead. My stomach pulled.

This is where it all began.

Though I'd resolved, stubbornly, to continue with my duties, my body was in a permanent state of numb. I knew deep down I was a good nurse, but no longer could I convince myself that I was a good person.

I moved to the side room to prepare the blood pressure machines and pulled out a stethoscope from the cupboard, winding the blue plastic tube tightly around my wrist. The stethoscope was a personal one that had my name etched onto the metal. A present from Mercedes to welcome me back because she said this moment was momentous.

I reached for the clinical wipes to give everything a good clean. Then I joined the other nurses for a quick handover. Thankfully, they were all from Platinum Care, so I could avoid questions, conversation, their endless staring. But when the handovers were done, I found myself searching the nurses' station once more. I wanted to see whether the key I'd hidden was still there, fixed with Blu Tack to the bottom of a metal cup of pencils.

I tilted the cup to the side. Sure enough, the silver caught my eye.

By instinct more than necessity, I visited the medical supplies room, surprised to find they hadn't even changed the lock. Of course, being short-staffed meant they'd cut corners.

I crept inside, standing there, observing the dark air around me.

My eyes adjusted and ran along the shelves, taking in the dizzying array of vials and mini boxes. To my left, the door of the controlled drugs cabinet. I felt unsteady on my feet, and as I turned, wanting to touch the door, I felt someone watching me in the shadows.

'Who is it?' I called.

Sandra appeared in the doorway. As she entered, her expression was sheepish, her left cheek lit up by the light streaming in from the window.

'I didn't mean to creep up on you,' she said. 'I just wanted to say, I hope you feel better. I can't imagine how difficult things have been with all that suspicion hanging.' She glanced stiffly around her. 'Should you be in here? I thought you weren't allowed . . . You know the rules have changed. At least two senior nurses must give approval for nurses to enter. Only Barbara and I can access this room and the controlled drugs cabinet.'

I nodded, but I didn't know whether I could trust her anymore. Not after what she'd said about me behind my back. And why was she even here, creeping up on me? Did she honestly have nothing better to do?

'I found the key on the front desk. I meant to return it. I was just checking it was the right one, that it worked in the door. Here, you can have it.'

Sandra nodded, unconvinced. There was an awkward silence between us as she took the key.

'Well, I came looking for you mainly because of the announcement,' she said.

'Announcement?'

'The date and time of the strike – between eight a.m. and eight p.m. on both the 15th and 20th December.'

'Oh?'

'The biggest strike ever in the NHS's seventy-five-year history. Can you imagine? The union have made it clear what we want. So now, it's time for action.'

The working conditions for nurses were shit. What was new? Still, it made sense for them to join forces, to make a stand, to speak out to the newly formed cabinet. Maybe then, the government might listen.

*Them.* I was conscious of my detachment.

'I'm aware,' I said.

'It's important we participate,' she said. 'Obviously, it needs planning, so we don't compromise care. That's what the press will focus on. They'll accuse us of being selfish, putting ourselves, instead of patients, first.'

'Sure,' I said, except I had other things to think about right now.

Sandra glanced down. 'So, you'll come?'

'Is it alright if I get back to you?' It was my first day back and I needed the work. But here Sandra was, already applying pressure.

Her face contorted, a look that said it all. I was no longer one of them. Most likely, I never was.

'Of course.' Sandra turned but then swung round. 'I don't suppose you could help. Peter Marshall, bed twenty-six. Needs his sheets changed. He's wet himself.' She scanned the room. 'I'm quite certain you're not supposed to be in here.'

I nodded, clenching my jaw. 'Sure. Be there in a sec,' I said.

*

'Sorry to disturb you. My name is Nina. We need to change your sheets.'

I stared down at the man before me, frail and thin. He was curled up on his side, pulling the edge of the sheet close to his chin.

'You should have come earlier,' he said. 'I'm sleeping.'

'You'll sleep more soundly in clean ones,' I replied.

I threw down a pile of sheets onto his bed. I placed my hands on my hips when he didn't move. I didn't know where Sandra was, which was typical. Probably with Barbara, telling tales about how she saw me loitering in the medical supplies room. I wouldn't put it past her, that stupid bitch. Some nurses had nothing better to do but snitch on others.

'Are you listening?' I asked. He opened his eyes. I could feel myself getting worked up. 'You need to let me do my job.'

His eyes widened.

Out of nowhere, Sandra appeared, glancing at me, then Peter, then back to me once again. 'Everything alright here?'

'We're fine,' I snapped.

Sandra was taken aback.

'I told her she should have come by earlier,' Peter scowled. 'She's disturbing me, I want to sleep.'

Sandra moved towards Peter, whispering. 'Sorry about this. It's her first shift back.'

I felt my face burn. Before I could stop myself, words fired out of my mouth. 'We're doing our best,' I said. 'We don't need your attitude when we're here, trying to help make you feel more comfortable.'

'That's a bit rude,' he quavered. 'All I'm saying is that

*now* isn't convenient. It's late. Like I said, I'm tired! Why didn't you come earlier?'

'Because you wet your bed *now*. It seems you can't control yourself. We need to change your sheets and wipe your backside down.'

I grabbed the sheets from the end of the bed and threw them open. But before I could do anything more, Sandra grabbed me firmly by the elbow.

'Nina!'

I saw her face, eyes throbbing, her cheeks scarlet. We stepped into the corridor.

'What's up?' I asked, rolling my eyes.

'What was that?'

'What's what?'

She appeared flummoxed. 'You're being *incredibly* aggressive. Go easy on him, okay? I know things are difficult, but you can't speak to a patient like that. It's appalling!'

*Appalling this. Appalling that.* She sounded exactly like Barbara.

Sandra fell silent.

'We're not the best of friends, are we? So, let's just keep it functional.' I bit my lip and glanced down at the vinyl floor. Stubborn, I felt like a child on the receiving end of a good telling-off. I once managed this woman. Look at her now.

'Maybe I was a bit hard on him,' I said. 'I'm sorry, okay?'

She fell silent. 'My God, Nina. What's happened to you?'

I shook my head. It was too much. I knew I was falling apart. What I did to him, to Leroy, could never be undone. Every patient I saw reminded me of *him*. That mixture of hate and disgust for myself.

'I need a minute,' I said.

I ran into the changing room and sat down on the bench, breathless.

Everything inside me felt terribly mixed up. None of my emotional responses were logically connected to my actions. I had killed a man, and in so doing, I had killed something in myself as well.

I settled my breath, breathing long and deep. Brushing myself down, I emerged after a few minutes.

I went to the kitchen to pour myself some water. My hands shook as I clenched on to my cup. The cold shocked my teeth as I drank. I didn't know how long I could carry on living as I was.

I felt a presence behind me.

'Welcome back.'

I turned. It was Barry. *Dear God. Not now.*

He stood there, larger than life, his stomach protruding, the keys on his waist jangling. He smelled of bread, like he'd just emerged from a bakery. But his face was worn; he appeared tired, as tired as I felt inside.

My heart quickened as a wave of panic and paranoia rushed over me. Barry's eyes said he had something serious to discuss with me.

I attempted a smile, keen to acknowledge his good intent.

'I was hoping to catch you,' he said. 'Don't suppose you have a minute? I've cleared it with Barbara.'

'Seems like I don't have a choice, then, do I?'

He gave me a look as if to question what I meant. Was I not happy to be here, my name cleared, given a second chance, even?

We moved to the family room, which appeared just as messy as I remembered it to be. I sat down, overcome by a desire to appear natural. I popped my feet on the table, leaving the TV playing in the background.

'Nina—'

I raised my hand. 'Can we make this quick? First day back and all. I'm rather busy.'

Barry glanced around him awkwardly, then turned, closing the door. He placed his hand into his pocket and stood over me like a giant.

'Is everything alright, Barry?' Having him just standing there was unsettling.

'I was wondering if you've seen Leroy Sanchez. Heard from him at all, since he left the hospital.'

My throat dried. I had to think carefully before opening my mouth. 'Why would I see him?'

Barry shifted the weight between his feet. 'It's just that he's missed a few key sessions and it's very unlike him.'

'I suspect he's busy stabbing people.'

'Nina, I'm serious.'

'So am I.' No good. I'd turned venomous. 'Why would *I* see him? Like I don't have better things to do. And where are you on Balraj's attacker? Any closer to arresting anyone?'

I pulled out a piece of gum from my pocket and popped it into my mouth. The strawberry flavour made my mouth water.

'I can't discuss that with you, Nina.'

I chortled. 'Course not. But you assume, because I was formerly accused by the hospital of certain failures in duties, that I'm a villain. Let me tell you, I did my best, Barry. I always did my best. Turns out there was corruption in this place, our CEO receiving backhanders. It is *disgraceful*. So, don't go asking me questions using that accusatory tone.'

Barry scratched his cheek. 'I meant nothing of the sort. You're acting strange, and dare I say it, defensive.'

'Is that your official observation, or merely personal?' I blew a bubble with my gum and popped it, a film of pink skin covering my lips. I peeled the gum off, stuffing it back into my mouth, chewing.

I walked to the door, gesturing to Barry that he ought to move out of the way. 'Look, I wouldn't worry. I'm sure he'll show up. As you can probably tell, I'm somewhat limited as a nurse now.'

'I did hear that,' said Barry, peering at me. 'Sorry to hear it. You'll be back to normal duties in no time. We'll always need good nurses, and you truly are a great one.'

I scoffed. 'And the police are great too,' I said sarcastically. 'What would this town be without you? Trustworthy, dependable. *Objective*. Keeping our streets safe. Always on the right side of the law, eh? Never colluding with criminals, because that would be terrible.'

Barry nodded, failing to catch my drift. The audacity and stupidity of him. I was about to leave, but he raised his hand before I could pass him.

'Nina, if you hear anything . . .'

I cut him a look.

I turned the handle of the door, slippery in my palm because of how much I was sweating. The TV was playing loud Indian music: shrieking notes from violins. The scene cut to a woman running.

# 33

We approached Christ Our Redeemer Community Church, arms looped under thick coats.

'This had better be good,' I said to Nikolaus.

He pressed his elbow down to lock me in. He lifted his collar and flakes of cigarette ash blew in the cold wind.

We shivered, noses frosted pink, determined to walk together confidently, regardless of whatever came next. Nikolaus took another drag of his cigarette. I tugged on his arm.

'Remember what I said. Just act normal. Don't ask too many questions.'

He nodded and we entered the courtyard, the smell of cinnamon and spiced oranges unfurling around us.

'I have no desire for attention,' he said.

'It's forty-eight hours since Barry spoke to me. Maybe things have moved on, but you never know.'

We passed a woman in a tracksuit and puffer jacket; I remembered her from the first meeting. She was talking to another woman. I remembered her too: red coat, lizard brooch. They opened a plastic bag, revealing an oversized Christmas stocking.

'Christmas, soon.' Nikolaus took a final drag of his cigarette and flicked the end. Unlinking his arm from mine, he rubbed his hands together.

'I can't think that far,' I said. 'Not with everything going on.'

This was how it would be. Constantly looking over our shoulders, questioning – sabotaging every good waking moment, every opportunity to be happy. Nikolaus kept his head down as we entered the church. The chairs were lined up theatre-style, greater in number than before. Neater, more formal.

'Just focus on what we do now,' I said. 'We've turned up here, just as we normally would.' It occurred to me how I was beginning to sound a lot like Barbara – pragmatic, functional.

Bernie Rogers stood to the side of the church hall and waved, then continued his conversation with three men surrounding him, presumably shopkeepers.

I moved to the snack table, dragging Nikolaus along, and poured a hot drink into two cups from the canister.

We sat down five rows from the back, but all I could think about was how everyone appeared to be watching us. Did they know something? Was there something about our behaviour or appearance that gave things away?

Farah was at the front, scribbling on her notepad, and I ducked my head.

The church filled up; I felt my body tense. Barry entered with three representatives I'd seen before from education, social services, Neighbourhood Watch. Pastor Oswald Otis was trailing behind them, waving to the crowd. They stirred as he passed.

Sheela was here too and I lowered my eyes, trying not to draw attention to myself. But it was too late. She had spotted me. She walked over and grabbed my arm.

'Did you hear? He is coming home.'

I was taken aback. 'That's wonderful. When?'

She leaned closer. 'Next week. But they do not have a wheelchair in Newgate. Can you believe it? We pay our taxes, but still, I must purchase one from a private company. He will need it for some time, maybe permanently. But let's see. I will take him to India for a second opinion. I do not trust UK doctors.'

I squeezed Sheela's hand. 'Any news from the police?' I searched her face, desperate for reassurance that Leroy was still somehow in the frame to justify my plunging a knife into him.

She shook her head. 'Nothing except to say that Balraj was caught up in the middle of fighting gangs. I do not expect much else. I hope you are okay now. It is terrible what they say about Newgate. I did not tell Balraj because it will upset him.'

I nodded.

A small bell rang, and Sheela left for her seat. I felt the heat pulse from my face as I caught sight of Grace near the front. She was wrapped in a thick scarf, left arm clutching a King James Bible.

I felt sick. If things weren't bad enough, as I turned, I spotted Manisha a few seats behind. Her face was a permanent scowl, her head wrapped in a plain white shawl.

Pastor Oswald Otis moved to the centre and grabbed hold of the microphone.

'Thank you, everyone, for coming here today. It really is incredible to see you all make such an effort. Before I begin, I just want to thank many kind members of the church for supplying today's cross-cultural treats. And, of course,

Derek. You are as sweet as the chocolates and cakes you've provided – alongside a generous donation.'

Everyone chuckled.

Nikolaus reached out his hand and squeezed my thigh. My eyes watered.

I leaned forward to listen to the two men seated in the row in front of us. The man on the left spoke first: 'Well, it's all a bit unexpected. His bright idea, apparently. Now, I'm not saying I don't think it's important to hear their side, but crimes have been committed. I've never heard of this process of bringing them in, getting them to talk about why they did it.'

The man on the right responded: 'Their way of asking for forgiveness, apparently. You know Otis. Somehow, God is always involved.'

'We're here to discuss the incident that took place in Civic Street,' said Pastor Otis. 'But it's important to understand, we're not here to judge. This is a gathering with restorative justice at its heart.'

The crowd hushed.

'It's a process that allows both sides to speak, to explain, how they see things from *their* perspective. It is the only process I know, aside from prayer, that might help this community heal after all the terrible things that have happened.'

Sitting there, listening to him speak, I felt a deep sense of remorse and regret.

'Does anyone wish to say anything before we begin?'

I swallowed and felt my stomach flip.

Barry looked up. 'I for one would like to say how deeply grateful I am to you for offering us this neutral space. We've needed a space to talk and to heal. This place is . . . powerful,' he said.

The crowd nodded. Pastor Otis smiled.

'We're about to bring them in, and you'll see they're just boys,' he said. 'Not the grown men they make out to be.' He paused, staring into the distance. 'It's important we give them time. Not many will listen without judgement.'

People shuffled in their seats.

'This is about learning and education,' said Barry. 'That's the purpose of this session.'

I glanced over to Grace and saw her nodding, dabbing a tissue over her eyes.

Pastor Oswald Otis sat down.

Quietly, three men filed in from a side door; their heads hung as they shuffled to the front. They appeared young and boyish. Each one wore hoodies and joggers. One of them wore a cap, another a leather jacket. The third had on enough jewellery for three people. None of them appeared to be older than twenty.

There was silence as they each sat down.

I leaned back in my chair. The tension grew and I scanned the crowd, feeling their questions hanging. I stared closely at the young men, and thought I recognised one of them. That one in the cap. I was sure he was with Leroy that afternoon, as I watched from the bus. As for the one wearing all the gold, he looked familiar too. Most likely he was with Leroy in the park that night, just before he was gunned down.

Barry and Pastor Otis gave one another a look.

'Thank you for coming today,' said Pastor Otis. 'You've been incredibly brave. Would you mind introducing yourselves, and then telling us, from your perspective, what happened that day on Civic Street.'

The young man in the cap straightened up. He twice cleared his throat. Even from where I was seated, I could see he was nervous.

'My name is Stephen,' he mumbled, glancing up at the ceiling as if wanting God to save him. 'Basically, yeah . . . none of us wanted to end up like this. In a gang. No one wants that life, but it just happened.'

The other two men nodded.

'We just got into it, starting from the bottom. Something to do. Some place to belong.'

'But why join SK in the first place?' asked Barry.

'What else is there? I—' His eyes darted.

'Go on,' said Barry. 'Take your time.'

'We was working our way up, yeah. Just like in a company.'

'We was there looking for a promotion,' said the man in the leather jacket. 'I'm Storm, by the way. Storm like thunder.'

No one appeared impressed by his swagger.

Pastor Otis urged the boys to continue after a momentary murmur.

'Each of us had our own reasoning. I'm Riz,' said the young man wearing all the jewellery. He stared down at the wooden floor, careful not to wind up the crowd as Storm had done before him.

'What happened on the afternoon of Monday 24th October?' Barry asked the question, twirling the wire of the microphone.

Storm shrugged his shoulders. Someone in the audience tutted.

'We was wanting to earn bank,' said Stephen. 'That's when someone said we should stain, because it would be easy, still.'

'What did you need the money for?' asked Pastor Otis.

A man in front shouted. 'He wanted to build a new hospital.'

The audience chuckled.

Pastor Otis raised his hand. '*Please*,' he said. 'Remember the importance of non-judgement.'

'We had beef with another gang, yeah . . .' Riz croaked, his nerves visibly kicking in. 'And like, we needed to bless it. That beef was over a missing stash of bud. We suspected someone from LH teefed it.'

'LH?' asked Pastor Otis.

'Mandem from Lyndon Hill. They didn't want us selling in their ends. But we still owed for the stash. None of us had that kind of bread to make it up.'

'But why target innocent people?' asked Barry, staring out into the audience. 'You can understand how much damage, and *pain*, your actions have caused. Your debt and dispute has affected everyone living in this town. And then the riot . . .'

'It was wrong, still. We know it was wrong.' Storm again. 'It was just to raise what we needed . . . but then LH heard about it, and it got big. Some of them saw the video on TikTok. They was bare jealous of the attention we was getting. Took it as a sign we were gonna come for them and keep selling in their ends.'

'You mean, a rival gang?' Pastor Otis, again.

The men nodded.

'You seem like intelligent young men to me. Were you aware of how much damage your actions would cause this community?'

'This our town too, yeah? We know there ain't much for us, here. Storm tried gettin a job but didn't pass the interview,' Stephen said.

'Would you be willing to take questions? I will be here to facilitate.' Barry appeared to grow nervous at his own request. 'People here want to know when this will end, with assurance that you'll put an end to the fighting.'

The men nodded reluctantly. Storm scratched his face. Stephen could not stop shaking his foot. Riz stiffened and would no longer make eye contact.

Nikolaus turned to me. 'They are brave to take such questions. Many here are wanting to kill them.'

'Stupid, more like,' I mumbled. While it was honourable that they'd come in, my mind still struggled with the justification they provided. All I could think was, *Balraj got stabbed and what for?* But then I remembered Leroy and the knife covered in blood.

Bernie was the first to rise. 'I get that things are hard. There aren't many opportunities, and for sure, there is prejudice. But an innocent man was maimed. You can't possibly justify what you did. How are we supposed to move on from here?'

Riz stood up, animated. 'That stabbing weren't us, yeah. We were there, but we didn't do it. It was the other mandem. They came in wanting beef, like I said. We was chill.'

*Chill.*

'And then we got framed,' said Riz. 'All the blame was on us.'

'But you *stole*. You made the video about the raid. Posted it on TikTok,' someone shouted from the audience.

'We was gonna stain a few phones, cigs, alcohol. Stuff we could sell. But when we had enough money, yeah, we was gonna dead it.'

Riz was up on his feet too.

'I don't believe them,' I said, leaning close to Nikolaus's ear. 'I know what I saw. I saw Leroy – he was part of it, stabbing Balraj.' But the truth is, I no longer knew what to believe. If Leroy was working with the police, he might simply have been observing and got too close, got caught up in the chaos. But still, looking at these men, allegedly helpless and innocent, I kept thinking they must surely understand why I felt the need to stab one of their own members.

Nikolaus nodded. 'I am with you on that.' He tapped my hand. 'One hundred per cent.'

If Leroy was an informant, they'd have had no idea one of their own was talking to the police. And so, if they suspected or found out, one of his own could have shot him. I stared at the men closely, wondering which one of them it was.

Sheela stood up and the crowd hushed. She was shaking, fidgeting with her hands. I held my breath, unsure whether I could watch what was about to happen.

'You people nearly *killed* my husband.' Her voice broke. 'His name is Balraj. He is in the hospital, his life ruined. He cannot work. He cannot walk. These days he no longer talks. My husband loved talking, once.' She sniffled, dabbing a tissue to her eyes. Storm and Stephen sat down, and so did Riz.

A woman in the audience wailed. Another soon followed.

It was all getting a bit heavy; my eyes were stinging; my chest grew tight.

Barry stood up awkwardly. 'I just want to make it clear that none of these men are accused or have been arrested in connection to the attack on Balraj. The perpetrator is believed to have come from the other side of town, from Lyndon Hill. Several suspects have already been brought in for questioning.'

More murmurs from the crowd.

'What is it you need to end this behaviour?' Pastor Otis intervened in a desperate bid to wrap things up swiftly.

'It's not like we don't want something different for ourselves,' said Stephen.

'Like what?' someone shouted. 'What is it you want in order to stop?'

'A job. Skills. We wanna earn. Some of us aren't safe. We can't get out from here, but we're not safe here, either.' Riz glanced round the church, perhaps searching for something.

'One of our mandem is missing. You know that, yeah? We know he's been hit. He hasn't been seen for days.' Storm trembled. 'This beef is getting out of control. We wanna dead it as much as you do.'

I squirmed in my seat. The audacity of them, when it was likely that one of them pulled the trigger.

'This is ridiculous.' A man walked out; three others followed behind him.

'No one can say Leroy was a shit person. He was part of

this community, raising money to do good with it. His mum is a good woman. Been a teacher all her life.' Stephen shook his head. 'So, none of you can say we ain't good for nothing and just low life.'

Grace raised her head and stood up. 'Thank you, son,' she said. 'Praise the Lord.'

'The problem is with some people making out they is good and really, they is causing trouble. That guy, Dev, is dead. That one in the hospital. It's a fucked-up case. But everyone knows he was dealin' for the opps. He sold us the stash and then we got robbed. No one knew we had it but him. Strange coincidence, if you ask me. But anyways, his story gets covering in the news, but Leroy, he's been gone for days, and jackshit has been said.'

There were gasps in the audience.

I was not sure what I was hearing. It was the first time I'd heard that Dev might have been associated with a rival gang, favouring one side, snitching on the other. I knew he was hustling to fund his music. But this was altogether different.

Manisha stood up. 'How dare you say that about my son!' she said. 'You've no right, no evidence. Dev had *nothing* to do with you or the trouble in town. No association with criminal gangs. That's you – all down to you!'

Grace also stood. 'I'm sorry for your loss. Really, I am. But my son is missing. Not one of you is aware or searching for him. He could be scared, alone, because of the reaction that young men like him receive in this town. Don't you see? These men are *all* our children. We owe them better.' She turned to Manisha. 'For God's sake, stop putting yours above all others. See this for what it is. Maybe you didn't know your son as well as you think you did.'

Manisha turned to Grace. 'Don't mix up *my* son with yours. My son was not a criminal.'

'You think your son is better than mine?' Grace laughed. 'Not according to these young men. Maybe you should think about that before running your mouth!'

More gasps, a few nervous laughs.

My mind raced through all the conversations I'd had with Dev. The weed, a bit of dealing, his concern over whether his own smoking had upset his stomach. Most definitely nothing about gang involvement.

Pastor Oswald Otis stood up. 'That's enough. We're closing this down.'

Manisha scoffed. 'This is a complete waste of time. I was willing to give it a chance until they mentioned Dev. Bringing down good people to make the bad ones feel better.'

She sat down, rearranging her shawl.

Storm shook his head. 'I ain't lying. He was dealing for the other side! He set us up. I'm not saying he wasn't smart. He was clever, like. Into music. He was gonna be big. But he ain't no good boy.'

I glanced at Manisha, about to stand up, the man next to her holding her down. Grace sat trembling.

'Know what I think?' Bernie was on his feet again, waving his fists, riling the crowds like a ringmaster. 'I think you lot started all this, so you can end it. You need to roll up your sleeves and sort this shit out with the other *mandem*, as you call it.'

I stared into the stained-glass windows, the hundreds of candles burning on the altar. Regardless of what they said,

I knew what I had seen that day from the bus. I'd seen Leroy there. But this talk of Dev left me wondering. Which one was bad, which one was good?

Barry stood up. 'We are intervening – applying the same principles of restorative justice to the other side. Our aim is to end this rift, to bring healing to this town.'

'Well, good luck with that!' someone shouted. 'And good luck finding that poor boy!'

I grabbed Nikolaus. 'Come on. We should go.'

I wondered whether God had played a sick joke on me, mixing up my sense of morality.

Reluctantly, Nikolaus stood up too, moving to the table to grab a bar of chocolate. He ripped open the wrapper as we shuffled towards the exit, several members of the crowd followed closely behind us.

Outside, I felt the bile rise at the back of my throat. I had suspected something like this before, but now, it was obvious that what I thought was good and bad was, in fact, in reverse order. I turned my face and caught a glimpse of the young men leaving the church. Stephen was being comforted with someone's arm around his shoulder.

'Did you understand what was going on in there?' I asked.

'I did not understand some of the language,' said Nikolaus. 'What does it mean?'

I stared down at the cracks of the pavement as we walked towards my flat.

'Nina?' asked Nikolaus. 'Is there a problem?'

I shook my head. 'It means things are now so much worse than we thought.'

# 34

Why had I ever bothered to return to the hospital? I no longer saw the point in being there when my notion of good and bad was jumbled.

I'd killed a good man. I may have believed he was bad, but it turned out he was good.

In Newgate, I tried to get on with my job, but Grace's voice haunted me each time I stopped. *My son is missing. Don't you see? These men are* all *our children . . .*

I weaved in and out of beds, tending to simple tasks, carrying out temperature checks, taking urine samples. But I refused to do bloods. The needle simply trembled in my fingers.

My eyes settled on an unassuming nurse, short with thick ankles, waddling heavy-footed. Purposeful, keen, full of energy. A stark reminder of what I once was. What it took to do this job well.

After a long shift, standing on my feet, I was about to collect a final urine sample from Premila Shah. She was a fifty-year-old fashion warehouse owner, a regular in West London's *Top Entrepreneur* magazine. Meant to be in for a day, but after visiting A&E, she'd complained of acute kidney pains and was transferred here after eight hours. She'd been kept in for overnight observation.

'You'd think they'd at least make these specimen pots a bit bigger,' said Premila. 'And I've been drinking all afternoon, but I think I can only squeeze a few drops.'

'We need more than a few drops,' I said. 'We'll be doing a CT KUB as well. That's scheduled in. I suggest you relax, pass as much fluid as you can in the meantime. Let me know when you're done. Or if you need help getting to the toilet.'

She stirred under her sheets.

'But why this urine test now? You did not explain it to me properly. You people need to explain things more, and not assume patients understand your procedures.'

I felt my patience wear thin like a veil. 'It's a test to see if you're passing any protein or other bacteria in your urine.'

'Oh?' Premila's face shrivelled, the corner of her eyes shaped like toppled question marks. 'Do you think it's something serious? Will I be okay?'

I'd been here before, with Manisha and Dev. I knew better than to promise miracle cures. 'We'll see,' I said coldly. It was all I could say. 'It could be kidney stones – that's what we're checking. But I do not have a crystal ball concerning your future health.'

Premila was taken aback.

I should have said something more appropriate, perhaps offering Premila a kind word or two as I waited for her to use the toilet and took away her cloudy urine sample. But every empathetic word was a strain. I was running on empty, my compassion expired.

At the end of my shift, just as the sun was rising through the windows, I gathered my things, leaving the ward quietly.

I waited for a bus under the shelter, one cheek of my buttocks propped on the red seat. My face felt tight and cold from the late autumn chill. In the distance, sounds of a Friday morning hummed around me. The bustle of excitement for the oncoming weekend, the promise of endless Christmas shopping, the start of festive merriment.

I saw the bus approach on the horizon and I fumbled for my pass. But just as I was about to get up, a white VW Polo pulled up onto the kerb. The passenger-side window lowered.

'Hop in. I'll drive you.' It was Farah.

I considered whether to run, but the bus was still some distance away.

'I can't park here . . . hurry!' Farah blew out a trail of smoke from her neon-pink vape. I glanced around me, checking no one from the hospital was near. I jumped in and buckled up, inhaling the scent of mint and watermelon.

'I'm trying to give up, but I can't,' said Farah. 'Hope it doesn't bother you.'

I shrugged, wondering what the hell she wanted. She'd already got a story out of me. As far as I was concerned, it was over between us.

She pulled away from the kerb, accelerating onto the main road. 'I was hoping to catch you, but you left the community meeting early.'

'It's not safe for me to be seen with you,' I said, stone-faced.

'I'll take us someplace private,' she said. 'A park.'

My stomach pinched as a flash memory of Leroy appeared. 'What is this about? I need to get home,' I blurted.

Farah pressed down on the gas. 'I'm working on a story.'

'You don't say.'

'Don't be like that. We got to a good place. I made good. Gave the evidence you sent me to Sid. You're reinstated at Newgate, so hear me out at least.'

I glanced out of the window, at the sensible houses flickering by, the front garden gates, the concrete drives. I wondered what it might be like to live a normal life.

Farah turned into a side road. I felt the wheels under my seat clunk as we drove over a pothole.

She parked up and switched off the engine. She took another puff on her vape and turned to me. 'You know that you can speak to me off the record, don't you?'

I stared into her eyes. I'd never noticed how dazzling they were. Flecks of almond around her irises, like sunflower petals. Her soft, silky hair framed her face elegantly.

I nodded.

'You'll know from the community meeting that a man is missing.'

'I am aware.' I felt sick; just the prospect of talking about Leroy was alarming.

'Grace's son. It's a travesty of justice, let me tell you, that it's only being reported *now*.'

'I was at the community meeting,' I said. 'It's clear he was involved with a gang. How do we know he's not on the run? He's probably hiding somewhere.'

'That might be so, but he's still missing. He's a son to a mother who is worried sick. I want to do a story on it, to highlight the unfair treatment. If it was a white man missing, he'd be on the front pages.'

I stared at my reflection in the wing mirror. Half black I was, but how I'd let that side of myself badly down. It was shameful that I'd considered myself different – better than Leroy. My fixation with Dev had been a representation of the good face I put on to be accepted. It was too hard being both.

'What's this got to do with me?'

'Leroy was treated at Newgate,' Farah said. 'Leroy Sanchez. At least, that's the name he went by. He was born Leroy Gibson.' She glanced at me. 'Do you know him, or have you heard his name? He was treated on your ward, according to my sources.'

'I can't remember all my patients.' I pinched the skin on my hands.

'But this one would have come with police protection.'

Of course they had been with him, not as escort to a criminal, but to keep their informant safe.

I didn't know what to say. I couldn't trust Farah. 'I'm bound by patient confidentiality,' I said.

'A man is missing!' She slammed her hands onto the steering wheel. 'Okay. Full disclosure. I *know* he was a patient of yours. At first, I admit, I couldn't believe it. First Dev. Now Leroy. You don't half attract them, Nina.'

I pulled at the handle, ready to jump out. I knew what this was – she was stitching me up.

Farah grabbed my arm. 'Listen. I just want to talk. I'm not accusing you of anything.'

I was breathing hard, fast. I caught sight of my face changing in the wing mirror. I glanced through the windscreen, watching a mother push a pram, stopping to unroll a rain cover.

She'd got me. She'd got me into a corner. I couldn't deny I knew Leroy, or that she'd done me a favour, passing the evidence I'd sourced on to Sid. But talking to her about Leroy would only lead to trouble.

'Like I said, patient confidentiality. I can't say anything

more than, yes, he was at Newgate. I treated him.' My heart thumped hard in my chest.

'Was there anything suspicious – *anything* to suggest where he might be now?' Farah's eyes flickered.

'I don't know anything,' I said. 'But a man like that is bound to have enemies.'

Farah scribbled something down, but she used funny symbols – shorthand. I couldn't understand a word of it. 'Is there anything you can tell me? Anything at all that might help? Grace is worried sick. We have a duty to report it.'

I flinched. 'I suspect the police know something. I would bet money on it.'

She sat back. 'What do you mean?'

'Maybe they knew him better than we think.'

Farah bit the end of her pen. 'Barry? Is that who you mean?'

'I've said enough already.'

'So, you *do* know something?' There was glee in her voice.

'Barry was close to him, that's all I know. He talked to him a lot on the ward.'

Farah's eyes lit up.

'Do you think Leroy is dead?' I asked. I tried to sound casual, but the panic was so intense, I could not hold it in anymore.

'According to my sources, he's been missing since Wednesday 9th November. He was last seen by his friends in Levinstone Park. After that night, nothing. Today is Friday 9th December – that's a whole *month* and nobody is doing anything.'

Farah's questions were too much. I needed to go. I needed to call Nikolaus. 'He's part of a gang. I would start there – with the *mandem*, as they call it.'

Her face screwed. 'There's stuff about him that people don't know. I was digging into him based on what was said in the community meeting. Turns out Leroy is not as bad as he appears. He won a scholarship at school. Won prizes for essays. He was bright and aspired to be a poet. Just goes to show, it's easy to judge a man and get it horribly wrong. That's what my angle is.'

My phone vibrated. I saw Nikolaus had sent me a text:

*Miss you. Many people have died. I must do a few extra shifts. xxx*

I turned to Farah. 'I gave you information about Newgate that landed *me* in the shit. And while you did me a favour with Sid, I'm still living with the consequences of an earlier version of your story. So please be clear about what you want, but know that what I'm offering you is minimal.'

Farah stared quizzically. 'Why are you so anxious?'

'I'm not.'

'You are.'

'Look, you'll get your story eventually. You always do. Knowing you, it'll be a bigger one.'

'Nina,' Farah averted her eyes. 'You're shaking.'

I blinked.

'Maybe it's PTSD – from reading one of your stories about me.'

I grabbed the door handle and pulled it hard. But this time, Farah did not hold me back. Instead, she started the car and wound down the window.

'I'll give you a lift back.'

'I'll walk,' I called.

'It's raining, Nina!'

I turned my back and ran.

On Oldfield Lane, I ran to my car and jumped in, desperately trying to catch my breath. I stared down at my veiny hands resting on the steering wheel, noticing how tired and worn they now appeared. Perhaps it was inevitable that the lives of abandoned children ended up being cursed. I sat there quietly in my car, concluding that Farah was right: it was only a matter of time before the truth surfaced.

The air inside the car was musty and stale. I could not bear to think of the stench of blood and the rotten fibres from the old carpet. Leroy was dead, but inside my car, the fan whirring, circulating the same deathly air, he still wasn't gone. I wound down my window. Even with it pouring with rain, I could *smell* him.

I started the engine and drove to Mercedes' flat. I didn't text her in advance.

Semis and shops whizzed past; they all looked the same. I eventually pulled up outside that familiar shabby front garden with its broken gate.

Switching off the engine, I glanced up at her window. The curtains were drawn. It was too early for her to be awake. I leaned back in my seat thinking of my best friend. I remembered what we were like in college: Mercedes the one who promised never to settle down, me the quiet one pushing hard, determined to make something of herself.

I fired her a text:

*I need to talk to you. I'm outside.*

But several minutes passed without her reply. I waited another thirty minutes and was about to leave. But then she responded:

*U should have told me u were coming! I'm not in –*
*sorry! With Sugar. She needed me to come over.*
*What's up? Nik already annoying you? LOL!*

I threw my phone down onto the passenger's seat.

I burned a man, that's what was up. The flames of his cremation now crackled inside of me. No matter how much I tried to move on, his death would be a stain on the rest of my life.

# 35

The following morning, after a difficult night tossing and turning, I got myself ready for my appointment with Frances. I clicked my mouse, and within seconds, I'd entered Zoom. I watched myself on screen, the dark circles beneath my vacant eyes, my cheeks pale and sunken.

I put myself on mute, grabbed hold of my phone and typed Mercedes a text as I waited for Frances.

*Let's meet in the canteen tomorrow. xx*

Frances appeared, her face filtered and warm, as if filmed in oil. Her hair haloed in orange light. She appeared fresh. The screen divided into two. I unmuted myself and switched on my camera.

'It's good to see you,' Frances said. She smiled, her teeth appearing yellow, her lipstick, bright pink. Her voice echoed like she was speaking into the drum of a washing machine.

'I really need this,' I said.

She took a sip of water. I heard her gulp. A knock of glass against wood as Frances placed down her tumbler.

I tried to settle, but inside I felt locked in a state of panic. I studied the room behind Frances to distract myself. It wasn't the elegant home office I'd seen before. This one resembled a hippie cavern, styled for a magazine. Rugs hanging off the walls, a table to the left with an oversized quartz lamp.

I glanced around my own studio and felt low. The place was a mess, once again, tin cans and cutlery in the sink. Dirty laundry spilling out of the basket. I was up and down, some days able to keep on top of things; other days, it was too much.

'When was the last time we saw one another? Let me see . . .' Frances fumbled through her papers; I couldn't see them on screen.

'Thursday 27th October,' I said.

'Ah, yes. I remember it now.' She'd located the relevant note, it seemed. 'That's quite some time ago. Almost six weeks.'

'Yes.'

'Why did you leave it so long?'

I was silent. 'I've had a lot going on,' I said.

'I see. Well, you're here now. That's all that matters.'

I bit the inside of my cheek.

'And how have you been feeling?' Frances glanced up, her eyebrows raised, her face full of optimism.

I felt my throat turn dry. I wasn't sure where I should begin. The last time I saw Frances, Dev had died, but now there was Leroy. 'A bit stronger,' I said; that much was true. *I am stronger, much stronger.* 'But I've been through the mill. I've been fired and reinstated. Seen death more times this year than during my entire career.'

*Also, I murdered someone . . .*

'It's never easy,' said Frances. 'In a climate like this, we can only continue as best as we can. I've heard about Newgate and what's been going on.'

I nodded. 'It's been . . . stressful.'

'It's terrible,' she said. 'Who would have thought?'

Frances glanced to the side of her, staring into the distance as if recalling our last conversation. 'We discussed writing and journaling, didn't we? How did that go, did you try it?'

I sighed. 'I wrote a few words, scribbles, scratches on paper. It meant absolutely nothing. I can't write. I'm just *terrible* at it.'

I heard the shuffle of paper once more. 'It's not a problem,' she said. 'You're not writing a novel. Simply processing your feelings. Don't be so hard on yourself. Maybe try writing yourself a letter.'

I felt a headache coming on. I needed water, two ibuprofen tablets, preferably with something strong like codeine. It would be easy to get up now, fix myself a glass. Possibly pour in some gin. One simple click of a button with my mouse and I could exit this session, even.

'It's important to get things out of your system,' she said.

Where would I possibly start? Nothing about my real problems could be discussed during the next hour.

'I'm in a dark place,' I said. 'It's not one thing, but a mixture of issues. I'm harder, angrier, than normal. It scares me. I don't recognise myself. I can't rely on my own judgement.'

I saw a flash of that night, the glow of the silver moon. The terror as we drove to the crematorium. That smell of dry wood and cinnamon.

Frances rearranged herself in her seat as I cupped my knees.

'The first thing I'd like to say, to reassure you, is that everything you're experiencing is normal,' said Frances.

'It is?'

'Perfectly. You are not a bad person.'

'I think I am,' I said. 'In fact, I *know* I am.'

'Well, let me tell you, you're not. You might not be an angel. But you're certainly not *bad*. I've seen too many good nurses break under the weight – the burden – of expectation, then be villainised. You are not expected to be perfect, no matter what society says. You're simply a woman doing a job that happens to provide a valuable service and is terribly underpaid.'

'Nursing doesn't feel the same anymore,' I said.

'And those feelings are normal,' said Frances. 'Your love and passion for the profession will return. It's one you chose for good reason. It's deep inside your heart.'

I wasn't sure whether I felt that way anymore.

'The fact remains, you still do it. You turn up to work. You're committed. You feel guilty because something outside your control has happened. It's part and parcel of the job. Those thoughts and feelings are natural.'

I struggled to listen.

'I counsel nurses like you each day. I am a good person, despite those dark moments I have. I am not a bad person for having, on occasion, an extreme feeling or thought that might suggest otherwise.'

But that was it, I'd passed that point. I'd crossed a line. I'd killed a man.

'The entire healthcare system is in turmoil. On top of an already difficult job, you carry that societal burden on your shoulders. Simply acknowledging that can be transformational.'

I wondered whether I should divulge now that I had no intention to strike with the others, holding up signs on the picket line, demanding fair wages and better working conditions. Right now, my problem was entirely different, far greater than anything going on in Newgate. I wasn't quick enough to interject because Frances continued.

'Tell me about some of the things you've been writing about.'

'Well . . . er . . . Let me see. I've been writing about Dev – or at least I *was* writing about him. A young man of twenty, who wanted to be a songwriter. I felt so bad that I didn't spot the signs. I know it wasn't my fault that he died, that in the end, it was the corruption, the messing up of blood results. But I didn't know that at the time. The thing is, I thought I knew him, but it turns out I didn't. Then we had a patient come in only a few minutes after Dev. His name was Leroy and . . .'

I felt myself clam up. I struggled to breathe. This story was complicated, and I was losing myself in it.

'I kept thinking . . . I can't choose between them. I can't *be* there, looking after both. I thought maybe that's why my mind divided them into good and bad, especially since the riot. But that was wrong. I'd got it wrong. Besides, I should have just been treating them, not thinking about anything else. Leroy was priority, I know that. But he was also not a very nice person.'

'Interesting.'

'And there he was, calling me, *taunting* me. If I could go back in time, I would have done things differently, I would not have judged so easily. I shouldn't have lost it.'

'But you did all the right things, despite your personal views. You prioritised within the circumstances and resources available. You suspended your own personal point of view to do what was right, observing the nurses' code. You acted without delay. You provided treatment, presumably, at his request and with his consent. You gave him the dignity he deserved. Most importantly, you put the patient in front of you first.'

Of course I did my job in the hospital. But I was no longer sure I'd observed the nurses' code as strictly as I should have done.

'How complex nursing is.' Frances looked up ponderously. 'You were not alone. Neither do you operate alone as a nurse. There are other nurses around you, other qualified medical professionals. It takes an entire team to take care of a patient. It's the same in every hospital.'

'Well, this one's in the papers for being particularly bad,' I said. 'But it's worse . . .'

Frances pursed her lips. 'I dread to think what the public inquiry will reveal.'

She glanced down. Though it was subtle, I knew our time was up. She was probably looking at her watch under the table, observing the minute hand ticking.

'I don't think I can do this anymore,' I said quickly. A last-minute attempt to keep her online for longer.

'These sessions?'

'Nursing. I thought it would make me feel valued because I was doing something good, after everything that happened to me. But it's impossible.'

'I am terribly sad to hear that,' Frances said, shaking her head. 'I never like to hear good nurses talk like that, especially given the crisis we're in, the one we've just had. We must create an invisible shield around us, a psychic armour, to protect us from pain. You're a nurse, Nina. You'll encounter death many times. I promise it will get easier, that you *will* find a way through the difficult choices you must make. You cannot allow one death to undo all your hard work.'

'But it's not just one.'

'However many there are. For every one death, there are a hundred lives you've helped. Never forget that.'

I felt an itch on my leg. It was crawling up my thigh. It moved along my arm like an ant, finding its way to my chest, neck and face. I was overcome by an urgent desire to scratch, scratch, scratch – clawing fingernails into skin. I wanted to draw blood, dig into flesh, just to relieve myself from it.

'It's worth exploring which aspect of death upsets you the most,' said Frances. 'Perhaps discuss it with your supervisors or write it down in your journal.'

I didn't think I could do that. It felt like torture.

'Then what?' I asked.

Frances hesitated. 'Burn it.'

My stomach flipped. 'Burn what?'

'Whatever it is that you wrote. Let the ashes of paper waft into the air like grey feathers in the wind. Let it all go. Release it. Rejoice in the freedom it brings. Then, re-energise yourself and your nursing practice.'

I felt sick.

'It's been good to see you, Nina. Please do take care of yourself. I'll email you a Doodle poll with a list of my next available slots.'

Frances waved. A black screen appeared. I closed the home page as the Zoom call ended.

*

That night, as I attempted to sleep, I recalled that night with Leroy in the park and began rewriting the scene. Instead of him calling out to me after he'd been shot, I pictured him already dead, me simply walking away with nothing more to do with him. A line had been drawn. That was the end.

I scrubbed that scene, then began mentally writing once more. I imagined what might have happened had I never entered the park. Most likely, I'd be sitting at home, watching TV, browsing a catalogue of clothes I had no money to buy, drooling over soft furnishings in an online magazine.

I sat up in bed and grabbed my phone. My face felt hot; my nightdress stuck to my back. The blue light lit up the room as I checked whether Mercedes had replied to my text.

Nothing yet.

I flopped back into bed, releasing a breathy sigh. Despite how conscious of my breath I was, it was impossible to unwind. I sat up again, throwing my legs to the side, and stood unsteadily to go fetch myself a drink. A strip of light glowed from beneath the front door. It illuminated the far end of the room, and I froze.

*Please God, don't let that be the police.*

Holding my breath, feeling it swelling inside me, I waited.

I heard a ruffle of paper slip under the door. The light turned off; footsteps descended the stairs. It was a woman, perhaps, her bangles jangling.

I flicked on the torch on my phone. I walked to the front door; there, on the doormat, was a brown envelope.

Seated on the edge of my bed, leaning to the side, I

switched on the lamp and ripped open the flap. The note inside was pink, handwritten:

*Tuesday, 10th December 2022*

*Dear Miss Nina,*

*I am home from the hospital and must manage some tasks. You have been a very good tenant, and I have always supported you. But now I am very sorry for bringing you sad news. Unfortunately, after this terrible incident, we are closing the Samosa Hut. We cannot stay here anymore. We do not feel safe. Everything we worked hard to build over the last thirty-five years in this country is gone. Sheela and I will be starting somewhere new. We are going to sell the shop and the flat you live in as well. We have a buyer who is very interested, but he is telling us he would like the flat for himself.*

*I am very sorry to tell you all this. I hope that you will find somewhere else nice to live. I cannot give you any help because of my condition. Sheela is busy and I don't want to give her more stress. Thank you for your understanding, please, I hope you will have dinner with us before you go. Because you have one month's notice, you must make sure the flat is empty by 31st January 2023. Because of Christmas holiday, you have more time. But it cannot be later than this. I am being reasonable so please do not leave anything. I know you will leave everything nice and tidy.*

*Mr Balraj Singh*
*Landlord*

# 36

This flat, once my home, would soon be gone. I didn't blame Balraj for his decision. I could, of course, understand. I thought about finding a cheap hotel, leaving my things in storage before devising a sensible plan. But a quick search online revealed that the cheapest room, £49 per night, was still more money than I had.

I searched rentaroomlondon.com. There, I found several listings for short-term lets not too far from where I lived. One listing caught my eye: already, seven likes. It was just on the border of Levinstone, close to Newgate Hospital. A lovely bright room available within a duplex flat. It boasted a shared living room, kitchen, and bathroom, all within a reasonable price. Facilities included a washing machine, microwave, high-speed Wi-Fi. But the thought of having to live in shared accommodation after all this time made me feel as if life was moving backwards. I remembered the Maple Tree Children's Home, the noises at odd hours, the screaming, shouting, the constant flushing of the toilet.

For the rest of the afternoon, I cleaned. I thought I'd try out one of those hacks I'd seen on TikTok using vinegar. I scrubbed down the cupboards with a damp cloth and upended the cutlery drawers. In the fridge, I removed each shelf, replacing them only when they gleamed.

Finally, on Monday morning, after a difficult night's sleep, I stepped outside for fresh air only to find the weather had turned strange. There was a flash of electricity in the sky, something salty on my tongue. The birds lasered through the air, circling overhead. After a few seconds, a flash of lightning struck, a rumble of thunder.

I grabbed my bag as the rain came pelting down. The wind whipped my hair and face. I lifted my collar to protect my neck. My eyes were firmly fixed on the pavements. I passed a news-stand to my left. The headline on the *Levinstone Gazette* was large and screaming:

*GANG LORD GONE MISSING*
*Full story on page 3.*

I stared at Leroy's photo. A shot of him standing beside an iron gate, wearing a hoodie and cap, a crucifix dangling on a thick rope chain. I frantically scanned the news pages as a shopkeeper ran out to check I wasn't stealing. The newspaper slipped between my fingers; a page fluttered and flew in the wind like a startled pigeon.

'You gonna pay for that? I can't sell that now, it's bloody wet!' I rummaged through my handbag and handed him a pound. Gathering the pages from the newspaper, I ran.

Inside my flat, I spread the soggy pages on the kitchen table to read:

*Local police are searching for missing gang leader, twenty-one-year-old Leroy Sanchez, recently discharged from Newgate Hospital after a stabbing. Reports indicate he's been missing since Wednesday 9th November 2022 and was last seen in Levinstone Park.*

*The Met Police has come under severe criticism for not taking Leroy's disappearance seriously because of his involvement with SK. His mother, Grace Gibson, made the following statement: 'I can tell you my Leroy is a good boy. No one joins a gang unless their life is a challenge. Despite what people think, Leroy did a lot of good. I urge the public to be open-minded because he is a young man with his whole life ahead of him. Don't judge a man until you've walked in his shoes. The police have a duty to find him.'*

*Leroy Sanchez was recently implicated in several local robberies on Bridge Road and Civic Street, as well as the stabbing of Balraj Singh, owner of the Samosa Hut, a crime for which he was cleared. Since his confirmed disappearance, several online posts have appeared in the Levinstone community forum, speculating that rival gangs might be responsible.*

I grabbed my phone and checked the forum:

Anon_2000
*They were always going to get him. He was running his mouth too much. That's what I heard.*

Flor23.90
*I heard the police don't care. They are responsible for delays and need to give us some answers!*

Rudra-12
*Who cares where he is? Good riddance!!*

Niamh5000

*He wasn't a bad kid. Some of us went to school with him. He was different. Had some values. Head screwed on. Not like most gang members. Poor lad. Hope he's okay.*

MFJJ90-2

*I just LOVE how people have got time to think about yutes when no one says crap about all the good people in the community working hard.*

X900_Fortune

*Seriously. Can we talk about the police? How can they not know where he is?!*

I placed my phone down and continued reading the news article:

*A talented all-round sportsman and gifted poet, Leroy attended Levinstone High School during his teens but also won a scholarship for creative writing and took classes at weekends. Anyone with any information should contact Levinstone Police.*

I stepped back from the table, stumbling. I grabbed my phone and called Nikolaus.

I whispered as he picked up. I was barely able to speak. 'Something's come up. It's important.'

'What is happening?' he said, alarmed.

'Leroy's in the papers. They're talking about his disappearance.'

He fell silent. I heard the blanket ruffle. 'Shall I come now?'

'We don't have time. Anything could happen. We've got to get our story straight.'

I heard him get out of bed. Something sounded like it had been knocked down. 'Tell me.'

I clenched my eyes closed.

'Remember this order: I went to the park and felt unwell, so I called you. You said you'd come over to see me but didn't have transport, so we agreed I'd collect you. I came home first, grabbed my keys. I drove to pick you up. We came back to mine and stayed here for the rest of the night. You left early to go to work the next day. Understand?'

'Understand. And the times?'

*The times. Of course. We'd need to be exact.*

I heard a knock on the door. I peeped through the peep-hole and saw Mercedes.

It was the last thing I needed. I hung up the phone and sent Nikolaus a kiss by text before I opened the door. She stood there staring at me sheepishly, then grimaced.

'What is it? I texted you, why didn't you respond?'

She brushed past me, moving into the flat. My heart raced. I thought she might know something – but it was far worse.

She moved to the window, staring out of the glass. A pigeon flew past and she flinched, placing a hand on the ledge to better balance herself. 'I need to tell you something, and I hope, I really hope, you'll understand.'

I sat down on the sofa, staring at her back. 'What's the matter? You're scaring me.'

She turned. 'I just want you to know that no matter what I tell you, it mustn't change anything.'

I felt myself stiffen. 'Mercedes . . .'

'Do you remember at Maple Tree, when we made a promise? We said we'd always be there for one another, no matter what.'

'I remember.'

'Sometimes life, and pressure, can make you do bad things.'

'Like what, exactly?'

'Do you remember that journalist, Farah?' Mercedes said.

I nodded, feeling uneasy. 'The one I sent information to . . .' *The one who stitched me up and still wanted more.*

Mercedes swallowed. 'Yeah. That one.'

'What about her?'

'She was asking me for information, too.'

I stared at Mercedes blankly. *What did you do?*

'She blackmailed me, told me that if I didn't give her information, she'd smear me.'

My head rushed. 'I don't get it.'

'I feel terrible. I've not been able to sleep. I knew I had to tell you because we couldn't continue like this, you not knowing the truth, me hiding it.'

I stood up and walked towards her, my face close to hers. 'What did you tell her?'

'She said the quality of care given to mothers in labour was a joke. Everyone needed to know about it. She said she had information on me and that to keep *my* name out of the papers, I'd need to give her a better story . . .'

I felt the room around me spin. 'You mean you—'

'I had to give her something!' said Mercedes. 'She's a journalist, you don't know what they're like.'

'Oh, but I do know, don't I?'

I stepped back, knocking my leg against the table.

'You understand, don't you?' said Mercedes, her voice raised. 'You're cleared now. You're fine. *Newgate* is under investigation, not you. It's not about you anymore. Things have moved on, so it doesn't matter, Nina . . . please!' She covered her face, sobbing. 'I know I shouldn't have done it. I'm *so* sorry, honestly, I am. I've been wanting to tell you for days.'

My face burned. 'You snitched on *me*? Your friend of so many years? After everything we've been through together?'

I watched her shoulders judder and then she wailed.

'That smear of me in the papers was based on information *you'd* given to that bitch, about me?'

*Snitch. It was all so reminiscent . . . I knew now how it felt.*

'It's not what matters now,' she said, her face damp. 'It's in the past. You got your job back. You need to focus on what's happening now.'

I grabbed her bag, throwing it into her face.

'Get out.'

'Nina, listen!'

I turned away. She was unreal, a traitor. I could hardly believe it.

She sniffed and picked up her bag. I heard the door close behind her and I sat down.

My head pounded as I tried to process what I'd just heard. I ought to have slapped her. Our promise. What a bloody nerve. I wanted a better explanation. I wanted to know why she'd sold *me* out when it could have been anyone else.

I got up and raced to the door, throwing it open to chase after her. But standing there instead was Barry.

He blinked and we stood there, staring at one another. 'Hope I'm not interrupting something, Nina.'

He had a small notebook and pencil in hand. The radio on his left shoulder crackled. He pressed a button to silence it and cocked his head inquisitively. 'Mind if I come in? I won't take too much of your time. Just doing the rounds.'

I swallowed.

'Presumably you've heard, now it's all official.'

'Leroy Sanchez,' I said. *What else could it be?*

Barry nodded.

I closed the door behind him, wondering where Mercedes had gone. I wanted to throttle her next time I saw her. But it hardly mattered. Here I was, about to be arrested.

'I read the story in the papers,' I said. *That fucking bitch Farah. She really was something.*

He stood by the window and glanced around him, to the sofa all neat with propped cushions, a blanket folded on the end, the counters, tiles, floors gleaming. 'Been busy, I see. Smells lovely and clean. Sorry to be here, making the place look untidy . . .'

I was about to agree with him, but I bit my tongue. 'What can I do for you?' I asked.

'Mind if I take a seat? I have a few questions.'

He didn't wait for me to answer and moved to the kitchen table.

I sat down on the sofa, nudging the blanket to one side; all I wanted to do was to lie down. 'You're wasting your time. Like I said before. I don't know anything.'

He turned, thumbing a finger over his newly grown moustache. 'Leroy Sanchez and you *do* have a connection.' He stared at me. 'I'd love to explore that a little.'

'I treated him as his nurse. Hardly a connection.'

Barry glanced down at the newspaper, flat open on the page about Leroy.

He sighed. 'Not many will be too motivated to ask questions, even after our meeting in church. But he's a good boy and I knew him well. His mother is devastated as you can imagine. We need to find him, Nina. I feel personally responsible.'

I scoffed. 'I'm sure you do.'

He shot me a look. 'We know he had enemies,' he said. 'But it's important to be fair. It's why I'm here.'

He opened his notebook. 'Did you see Leroy at all after you treated him – like outside Newgate Hospital?'

I opened and then folded the blanket next to me, to give myself a couple of seconds to compose my answer. 'Possibly,' I said. My hands began to tremble. 'I saw him in the park. I remember it now.'

'Park, when was that?'

Barry sat up. I instantly regretted saying it. But I knew I wouldn't be able to lie about it. His gang of cronies had seen me there that afternoon and most likely told him. I watched Barry scribble something down in his notebook.

'Can you remember the date?' asked Barry, his voice dry and quieter. He was thinking.

Of course I knew. How could I forget? 'Not sure. Possibly the Wednesday or Thursday, I think . . .' I stood up, moving to the calendar stuck to the cork board. I ran my finger over the days. 'Mmm. It was the ninth. I remember it now. I was fired. That day, I wanted to clear my head. I remember it now.'

He nodded. 'Time, roughly?'

'Possibly around four. I went for a walk initially and ended up at the park.' *Times. I hadn't managed to confirm the times. Nikolaus and I urgently needed to get our stories straight before Barry got to him.* 'I left here around four, so that means I must have seen him around thirty minutes later, say four thirty. He was with his gang, in the distance, across the green. I walked straight past them.'

'I see.' Barry scribbled some more. 'Did you talk to him at all?' he asked.

'No.'

'You're sure? It's important since the ninth is the day he went missing. You may well have been the last person to see him.' He stared hard at me. I felt something pierce through my heart. He knew – or had seen something. Maybe CCTV or something else. I thought there were no cameras in the area. But could I be a hundred per cent sure? It wasn't worth the risk. I decided to change tack.

'Hang on. I do remember . . . we exchanged a few words. But only a few. Apologies. It was so minor I almost forgot about it.'

Barry seemed reassured that this revelation had confirmed his suspicions all along. But I kept thinking about Mercedes. I'd trusted her with my friendship when all along, she'd stabbed me in the stomach.

'How long was your conversation and what did you discuss?' His face did not flinch. I struggled to concentrate.

'Five minutes, tops,' I said.

'What did you talk about, Nina?' His tone turned suddenly aggressive.

'I just asked him how he was, that's all. He told me he was recovering well.'

'That's all?'

The speed of his questions was making me nervous.

'That's all.'

'And that took a full five minutes?'

I shrugged.

'Is there anything else you want to tell me, Nina?' Barry glanced up from his notebook. His behaviour was so true to a TV crime drama it seemed almost comical.

I hesitated, attempting to suppress nervous laughter. 'What do you mean? I'm not the one lying.'

He stared at me. 'Meaning what exactly?'

My lip trembled. 'You knew him best. Why ask *me* so many questions?'

He looked down, shaking his head, as if he had resolved not to rise to any of my comments.

'Let's stick to the questions, shall we? Where were you later that night?'

I glanced up at my calendar once again. 'I was at home, why?'

'Can anyone corroborate that?'

'Sure.'

'Who?'

'Nikolaus, a porter – mortician – from Newgate. When I returned home, I called him.' This was a mistake. I knew immediately it was a mistake. I was supposed to say *I rang him from the park before arriving home. Idiot, idiot!*

'Can Nikolaus corroborate your story?'

'Sorry, I called him from the park, on the way home. I was feeling unwell, and he said he'd come over but needed a lift. So, I went home, then collected him. And we returned here and stayed here all night.'

'I see.'

For a second, I felt proud of myself for the neat correction.

Barry glanced down at the carpet, turning something over in his mind. 'What time did he leave?'

His interrogation was beginning to grate, the quantity of his questions, utterly exhausting. 'I don't know. Early the next morning . . . around six, I think.'

'Mmm.'

I did not like the sound of his *mmm*. I could no longer trust myself to remember essential details. I wanted water, something to ground myself.

Barry nodded to himself, and his face screwed a little around the mouth. 'It's important you share any information that might help inform our investigation, Nina. Withholding information is a crime, also.'

God, he had a nerve. 'I don't know what you're implying. I've told you everything I know. I've told you the truth. Do you even know what that is?'

Barry nodded like he might be satisfied. I let out a long, silent exhale, relieved it was all over. But his eyes swept around the room and he continued talking. 'Cosy little place you've got here, Nina. I hear the samosas downstairs are amazing.'

I did not deign to offer him a response. I felt so sad, just then. I was thinking of Balraj, how I'd be leaving him. The state of my friendship with Mercedes. What a way for things to end.

Barry straightened his back. 'Well. I've got everything I need. That's all my questions for now.'

I had a strong desire to run to the toilet to be sick. But I stayed where I was, moving to the door as Barry made his exit.

He turned the handle of the door, then swung round suddenly. 'Just one more thing.' He stared at me pointedly. 'Dev's death. You're currently no longer part of an investigation, but your duties have been altered, yes?'

I felt the iron guard rails inside me lift. 'I did nothing wrong, Barry. It was an unfortunate event. We were all devastated by it and I needed support. So yes, adjustments have been made. The real crime is the corruption that took place at Newgate.'

'I see.' Up close, I saw his front teeth were a little crooked. 'Best be on my way. Thanks for the information.'

I nodded, disbelieving, trying to figure out whether he was just being sarcastic.

He took a few steps down the staircase but then turned back once more. 'I'm off to the vigil tonight,' he said, 'it's for Leroy. Eight o'clock in the town square. Perhaps I'll see you there?'

That's when I knew – he was withholding something. A vital clue, a mistake I'd made. He most definitely had something on me.

He waved, his hand gripping the banister as he climbed down. 'Everyone will be there to show their support.'

I closed the door, pressing my back to it, my breathing fast, shallow, sweat dripping down my spine.

In my flat, by the window, I watched Barry step onto the pavement, glancing left, then right. The crown of his head bobbed as he trotted, at speed, down the road. He appeared to be a man feeling pleased with himself. Turning the corner at the end, he disappeared.

I flopped onto the sofa, knowing that there was no way I could avoid the vigil now. If I was absent after he'd mentioned it, he'd assume I was hiding something.

I grabbed a fistful of hair, pulling at the end. Snatching my phone from the table, I thumbed Nikolaus a text:

*There's a vigil for Leroy. It's tonight at 8 p.m. in the town square – 5 mins from me. Can you make it? We must go.*

I was careful not to write anything more incriminating. Nikolaus fired a text back.

*Ok. I come.*

# 37

The air was crisp against my cheeks. Glancing up through the mist, I could just about make out the town square, the parade of shops lit up with Christmas lights twinkling in the dark. Disused commercial properties with fallen bins. A frozen fountain in the middle. Chestnuts spat and crackled on roasting pits. I passed a concrete bench, armrests covered in pigeon droppings.

The cold cut into my skin. My body moved but with a second's delay. Something felt horribly off balance, electrolytes fizzing before running out of spark.

I felt terribly alone and abandoned, the sense of everything I'd ever known and trusted, dissolving. Crowds spilled into the middle of the square. Some carried flickering candles. Children clutched bags of chips and chicken sticks, grabbing their parents' gloved hands.

This was a town I loved, a town I'd miss. A town I thought would be forever a part of me.

I rummaged in my bag to check my phone. Nikolaus had sent me a message, which said simply: *5 mins*.

Nothing from Mercedes.

I moved to the side where a family gathered, catching sight of a woman with thick, braided hair, twisting a scarf around her neck. It was Grace, wearing a grey coat, standing with two men, their faces angry yet grief-stricken. A young woman walked to the front carrying a microphone.

A cable trailed along the wet concrete.

A speaker pierced the air with a moment's feedback; I winced at the high-pitched sound. The murmuring crowds took that as a cue to quieten and settle down.

Grace moved to the front, stepping closer to the microphone. She dabbed a tissue on each eye, then paused, taking a moment to compose herself. 'It means so much to me that you all came,' she said.

I skimmed faces in the crowd, searching for Nikolaus. When I didn't see him, my nervousness grew.

'What you see before you is a mother searching for her son. No matter what they say, no matter what's happened in this town, I know Leroy is a good man. To anyone who knows where he is, please bring him home.'

The rush in my head was so intense, I struggled to maintain my balance.

'I know in my heart he is alive and well somewhere,' she said. 'He is so full of energy. The kind of man that can get out of any situation. Sure, he is not perfect, but he did so much good. The police know that. But those are the stories about him we never hear.'

I felt a tap on my shoulder and, to my relief, it was Nikolaus. I grabbed hold of him and drew him close. He clutched my arm but failed to meet my eye, conscious we were being watched.

'Please, if anyone has any information that might help, I beg you to show yourself.'

In the distance, a swarm of boys approached in black hoodies. They did not carry candles. I felt the skin on the back of my neck prickle. A man, part of the group, broke free and stepped forward. His face was covered with a red bandana. He shouted, 'He was a snake! We know what he did! He was chattin' to the police!'

Grace ignored him.

'I brought up my son on my own. In the absence of a father, I taught him to be his own man. Whatever you think he is, he doesn't deserve *this*. He could be in danger, and we must find him.'

Barry stepped in with a line of police, ready to pounce.

'Don't you see? He is one of us. He is my son!' Grace began wailing and had to be carried off. Staggering, she leaned onto a man's shoulder.

Many in the crowd buried their faces into tissued hands. But then another man shouted. 'You've had your chance to speak. No good came from you lot being here. You've brought nothing but trouble and violence. So now we say it's time for you lot to piss off and give our town back.'

The crowd erupted. More men appeared, gathering and thickening their band of support. They were mostly white and wore white sweatshirts, the words 'Reclaim England' splashed on the front. Their faces were half covered with scarves.

'These streets are ours,' one shouted.

'We're not racist or violent but this can't go on,' said another. Someone threw a bottle. It landed with a smash. Before we knew what was going on, more bottles flew past. The police came rushing out.

I grabbed Nikolaus, pulling him to the side, watching in disbelief as the police formed a line separating the men from Reclaim England from those in hoodies. Black and red bandanas mingled.

Each side spat and cursed, showing heft and muscle. This was the real implication of the town's degeneration into street violence: the extreme far-right entering the cracks that had formed within our community.

I turned to Nikolaus. 'Listen to me, Barry is closing in.' We stood at the back of the crowd, just outside a vape shop. Despite what was going on, I *had* to stay focused. 'He's been round, asking all sorts of questions about Leroy's disappearance. This is fucking serious.'

'What does it mean?' asked Nikolaus. 'What did the police ask?' Nikolaus was shifting on the spot. He unzipped his jacket and pulled out a cigarette. We moved further to the side, just in case another bottle landed near our heads.

'He wanted details of our movements that night. So Stefan must keep his mouth shut. We need to be precise.'

'Shall we leave?' he said. 'Look at this. It is terrible. I see this in Germany. I did not expect to see it in UK.'

'Don't see why we should,' I said. 'Besides, it will look suspicious.'

'But this crowd is angry,' he pleaded. 'It is not safe for us.'

'I'm not safe,' I said. 'You'll be fine.'

Nikolaus scratched his head and lit up his cigarette, sucking hard on the end. 'What did you tell Barry?' He released a long, smoky breath.

'I said that we were together all night like we discussed.'

'Maybe it's better I come to your place. Barry must see us together. For sure, we cannot stay here.'

The police attempted to contain the crowds, talking to

them, trying to calm them down. But the men continued to spit their vitriol. A riot van arrived. More police stepped out of the back carrying giant screens and batons. Their attempt to assert their authority, to reassure the public that their priority was to protect them. All the while, an undercurrent of menace from the hooded men was rising.

By now, most of the town's ordinary people had disappeared, disgusted and fearful of the far-right and gang presence.

I stared at Nikolaus's pale face, then at the crowds. I felt like an outsider.

Nikolaus grabbed me, holding me tight. All I kept thinking was that I'd failed to see the dangers of choosing a side. Were Leroy and I any different from one another? Why had I cast judgement?

'I've just been served notice,' I said. 'Everything is a mess. I'm having to move out, on top of everything.'

'What?' Nikolaus looked down. 'When?'

'The letter said by January 31st.'

He squeezed me tighter. 'We stay together. Do not worry. I'm here. We will get through this.'

My heart skipped and I pulled my eyes away as they filled. I watched people taking turns to comfort Leroy's mother.

The police now had Reclaim England surrounded. One of them tried to talk sense into a man, tall and thin, who appeared to be their leader. He might have been a local, hard to tell. His face was covered. But there were no other local faces I recognised. Many of them seemed to have come from nearby towns, to help make up numbers. I wondered if the police might be cutting a deal. It would be just like them: different causes, but the same tried-and-tested methods.

'I should never have got you involved,' I said. 'But you were the only one I could trust.'

He squeezed my shoulder. I was about to continue, to drum it into him that just because I *did* involve him, it didn't mean we had to stay together. He was free to leave and never look back. Look what was happening, didn't he see? It was unfair to cage him. But then he spoke.

'I love you, Nina.'

The wind whipped my face and took my breath away.

'I love you, too,' I managed. I was about to tell him more – that being with him made me feel complete, that despite my fragmented parts, he was the one – the only one – that made me feel whole. But in the corner of my eye, I saw Barry approaching.

'Fuck,' I said. 'Now what?'

'You must be Nikolaus,' said Barry, standing next to us.

'I see you in the hospital, but we never talk. Nice to meet you,' Nikolaus replied. He choked up and cleared his throat.

Barry nodded, scanning the crowds. 'Terribly worrying, all this,' he said, throwing me a glance. 'The trouble is, when a community divides itself, it attracts the worst kind to fill in the gap. I only hope Leroy's found. This was supposed to be a peaceful vigil to offer his mother support.' He shook his head.

'You knew him well,' I said.

Nikolaus lit up another cigarette.

'A man like that is hard to miss,' said Barry, cocking his head to one side. 'He's a man with many secrets, I'll give him that. But he's someone's son, much loved and missed. He's had a hard life, like many of us have. We owe it to his mother to protect him.'

'I hope they find him,' I said. I held my breath and said nothing more. I watched the crowds as they began to finally disperse.

Reclaim's men stuck up two fingers at the crowds. Men in hoodies threw beer cans. 'Scum,' they shouted. 'We'll kill you when you're alone!'

'I hope they find him, too,' he said, staring at me. 'We've made an arrest. I thought you might like to know that.'

'Arrest?' I almost choked.

Barry leaned closer. 'A rival gang member, Lyndon Hill. Based on intelligence we had. The kind hard to get – from the inside.' He glanced down. 'We have someone in custody, due to be charged with stabbing Balraj.'

'Oh? That's great. You didn't mention that before.' My voice wobbled. I tugged on Nikolaus's sleeve. 'Did you hear that Nikolaus? They've found the man who stabbed Balraj!' My heart was thumping hard.

'Not a man, a woman,' said Barry.

*A woman?*

'Well, I'd better be off. This investigation is hotting up. So much changing by the hour!'

Barry moved to the line of police as men from Reclaim England spat on pavement slabs and swaggered off. The other boys in hoodies divided and dispersed, red and black bandanas moving in opposite directions. But this confrontation was only the beginning. I knew there would be more.

I caught sight of Manisha and, before I could duck, she

approached. She appeared softer in the dark, the whites of her eyes clearer and shining under the flickers of street light.

'Nina . . .'

I didn't know where to look. My head was still spinning with news of the woman arrested over stabbing Balraj.

She placed her hand on my arm. 'I just want to say, I'm sorry. I know it wasn't your fault. What I said was unacceptable.'

I glanced up at her face; I felt my eyes sting, something inside me break. 'I'm sorry for your loss, really I am.'

She bit her lip, as if unable to say anything more. She nodded before walking off, leaving me standing numb.

The police stood on guard, preparing for a possible return. Barry was talking to one of them.

I grabbed Nikolaus, and he placed a hand upon mine. We walked quickly towards a narrow, unassuming alleyway next to an 'open all hours' chicken shop.

'Stick to the story, no matter what happens, no matter how much pressure they apply.' My voice croaked. 'On the ninth, I called you around 5.15 p.m., then collected you at six from work. We went straight to mine. You left the next day at 6 a.m. Those are the timings.' I glanced around me, left, right, to be sure that no one was listening. 'You must remember that.'

'I am a professional,' Nikolaus said, almost jokingly. 'You do not need to worry.'

'Repeat it.'

'Five fifteen call. Collecting six. To your flat. I leave at six the following morning – after some quality time.' He grinned.

I flinched. 'It's not funny, Nikolaus.' I covered my face. I knew he was nervous as hell, that his laughing was just his way of dealing with it. 'FaceTime me if anything happens . . .' But I didn't wait for his reply. I pulled away from him to get out of there as quickly as possible. I was aware that if the men from Reclaim England returned, I would be one of the people of colour they would beat down.

I walked towards the crossing to my flat, hoping this would all go away. I was being naïve. This was a murder investigation.

But still, looking back now at this final moment, I so wish I had told Nikolaus just how much he meant to me.

# 38

Approaching Newgate Hospital, I no longer felt like I belonged. I glanced at the nurses lining up on the picket line, simply passing them like a floating ghost. My eyes were firmly fixed on the ground. In the ward changing room, I threw on my scrubs, scraping my hair back tightly into a bun.

Reggie was cleaning the corridor. Still here. Consistent, dependable. Had he not allowed me to enter Richard's office that night, Dev's death might still be a mystery.

He waved the moment he saw me emerging from the changing room.

'Nina! Ready for another busy night?'

I shrugged.

He still had a pencil snuck behind his ear.

'Do you write poetry, Reggie?' I asked, approaching him. 'Only, some people say you do.'

He smiled. 'I do.'

'I'd love to hear it. Read me something.'

His face lit up. 'Since you're asking . . .'

He leaned his weight on the broom propped upright in his hands.

*'There are too many pigeons in this broken part of town.*
*Talcum powder feathers, fallen, dirty, crowns.*
*They fly into the ghettos; they know where they belong.*
*Flesh torn and bleeding, we hear their sorrowful song . . .'*

I nodded to the floor, taken aback by the depth in Reggie's words. 'That's great, Reggie, really great.'

He smiled. 'No matter what shit goes on in here, I have the words for it.' He chuckled, the tip of his brush like a microphone stand swinging between his hands.

The ward was empty and hollow. Patient service, transactional. Tension hung in the air, knowing the nurses were unhappy. Holding placards outside, they shouted for acknowledgement of their efforts. Better pay at five per cent plus inflation. Better working conditions – the difference between eating packet-only and fresh and healthy food.

I heard a patient call from behind a set of blue curtains.

'Oi, nurse! Can you wheel over a TV? I'm desperate to watch something. It's so boring in here.'

I approached bed fifteen. A young man no older than twenty lay on his back wearing khaki pyjamas. He had one knee raised, the other leg in a cast, a stray arm bent behind his head.

'I'll find one for you,' I mumbled. 'What do you fancy watching?'

He scanned my face, examining my features as if trying to figure me out. This young, entitled man, seemed intent on testing my patience.

'*Undercover Cops.*' He grinned. 'My favourite.'

I was about to turn, but he called out to me again. 'Why is it that I feel worse in here than I did before? Nothing ever happens around here, know what I mean? I'm stuck in time just lying here.'

I feigned a smile. 'You'll soon be out,' I said. 'And this –' I turned, throwing an arm in the air '– will all be a distant memory. No one wants to remember their time in a hospital, do they?' Something about that very thought brought sadness.

'But you'll still be here,' he said. 'Seriously, who would want this job?'

I swallowed hard.

I located a TV on wheels next to bed thirty-three, where Leela was recovering from an overdose of one hundred and twenty-three ibuprofen tablets. I rolled the TV towards him, unwinding the long cable, slamming the plug into the socket. I returned to the front desk, my footsteps heavy.

The phone rang and I glanced around me, unsure what I should do, whether I ought to take the initiative and pick it up – whether I was even allowed to. I was about to answer, but before I could, Barbara ran towards me, grabbing hold of the receiver. She mumbled, typing onto the keyboard with one finger. I walked off as Barbara placed the phone down. She called out to me.

'A new one coming up. Daisy May. Eighty-one years old. Will be here in five minutes. Broken arm.'

'Got it.' I straightened myself and rubbed my hands with sanitiser.

'Oh, and Nina—' Barbara said.

'Yes?'

'Chin up. You're going to be okay. We'll always need good nurses.'

I stared down at Daisy. Her face pale, covered in pink blotches. 'Hello,' I said. 'My name is Nina. I've been assigned to look after you.'

'I don't want to be any trouble,' she said.

'You're in hospital. You're no trouble at all.' I stood at the end of Daisy's bed, flicking through her notes.

I saw the apprehension in her eyes. She clutched her sheet, gripping it so tightly her knuckles turned white.

'I don't want to be here,' she said. 'I was fine at home. I can still move around on my own. I just had a fall, that's all. I don't suppose you've seen my poppy anywhere, have you?'

'Poppy?'

'Do you think they took it?'

'I can ask,' I said. 'Do you mind if I take a little look under your gown? I want to check the side on which you fell.'

She stiffened as I drew the blue curtains. The air between us grew more intimate.

'Why would they take my poppy?' asked Daisy. 'Only just bought it last month.'

'I'm sure it's around somewhere.'

I lifted her gown, my heart sinking when I saw the blue bruise the size of a handprint slapped on her lower back. I replaced the gown, rearranging the blanket. 'I'll see if I can get you some heparinoid cream,' I said. 'I'll be back in a minute. Do let me know if you need anything else.'

By the time I returned, Daisy was calm, more settled.

'I know I shouldn't be here,' she said, staring up at the ceiling. 'I know they want me out. I don't want to be any trouble, but I haven't got anyone to call.'

'We're making enquiries now,' I said. 'Please don't worry.'

'What's going to happen?' Daisy's voice was barely a whisper.

I pulled up a seat and sat down beside her. 'Well . . .

we'll speak to social services, and they'll come in and talk to you about a care package that involves adaptations to your home. We know you've been having a few accidents lately. We can't take any more risks. You understand that, don't you?'

Daisy closed her eyes and nodded. 'I was like you, once. Full of energy, always bouncing around. The years go by so quickly.'

I felt a lump in my throat. She turned her face, staring at me.

'Don't waste your good health,' she said. 'It goes before you even know it.'

I bought her a poppy from the hospital shop, which was not easy since Remembrance Day was last month and they didn't have any more – except the last one – in stock. That evening, as I prepared to leave, a porter wheeled Daisy away and I thought of Nikolaus.

'Hang on!' I called.

The porter turned and stopped at the door.

'I just wanted to wish you luck.' I pressed the poppy into Daisy's hand.

She stroked the red paper petals in her palm, then brought it close to her chest. 'Reminds me of my dad. He fought in World War I,' she said. 'He said it was the proudest thing he'd ever done, fighting for a Great Britain.'

I watched the porter wheel Daisy out of the ward and stood there for a while as the doors closed. In the changing room, no longer bothered about climbing out of my scrubs, I grabbed my coat but was taken aback when Mercedes entered.

'I'm glad I caught you,' she said quickly.

My defences rose. 'I've nothing to say,' I spat.

'Look, I know you're angry—'

'Me, angry? What the hell do you expect?'

'I'm sorry!' she cried. 'I know I fucked up, but we can't hold grudges now. I came as quickly as I could.'

Mercedes appeared different, her eyes wild and alive, her hair fuller and dyed red. It was like she was on fire.

'I'm due back on the picket line but I had to see you,' she said. 'We can't leave it like this.'

'I think we can.' I turned my back.

'I know you're scared. But no matter what happens, we said we'd always be there for one another. So, I'm here, when it matters. Just like I promised I'd be. I'm not perfect, but I kept my word.'

I stared at Mercedes blankly. She made no sense. It was just like her to get dramatic over the most trivial of things. All this, to downplay what she'd done.

Her face contorted. 'Oh God. You don't know, do you . . . ?'

'Know what?'

She covered her eyes.

'I don't have time for this,' I said, and began gathering my things.

Mercedes sat down on the wooden bench, her back bent, chest heaving. 'I feel terrible,' she said. She tilted her face. 'But I did tell you, didn't I? I *told* you he was weird.'

'What are you talking about?'

She glanced up and swallowed. 'The police were here. They've arrested Nikolaus. Something about . . . murder.'

# 39

Tears disintegrated on my cheeks as I ran before the police could find me. I scanned the glittering road as a flash of shoppers hurried along the pavement.

In the distance, that familiar red bus. I stopped, breathless, holding out my arm. The driver stopped and the doors opened. I staggered onto the bus, desperate to talk to Nikolaus. I needed to find out what happened. I needed to know what he'd said. All I wanted, in that moment, was to hear his voice again.

The bus pulled away from the kerb. As I sat there, I pictured the police storming into the mortuary. Nikolaus falling to his knees, them wrenching his arms behind his back. I hoped he'd said something to protect himself. Ideally, nothing to incriminate me, though I would understand if he had. None of this was his fault. If I could take it back, I'd do anything to save him.

In my flat, I frantically scanned the room. It appeared to me like an unfamiliar space inhabited by a stranger. A sense of abandonment washed over me as I hunted for my small rucksack, stuffed at the back of my closet. I grabbed whatever I could. Two pairs of joggers, five clean T-shirts. Rifling through a pile of towels, sniffing which ones were clean, I grabbed my favourite one, along with grey socks and a pair of thick tights. My first thought, to catch the Tube to Westminster, to hide in a cheap hostel.

I felt a stab in my stomach thinking of Nikolaus, knowing that he was most likely being interrogated by the police. I knew he'd try to stay strong under pressure but the thought of how they might treat him made me feel sick.

My phone rang, I saw Mercedes' name flash. For a second, I hesitated, but then I answered.

'Where are you?' she asked.

There were crowds in the background, cars beeping, whistles blowing.

'I'm at home.' The phone crackled.

'Look, I'm really scared right now. People at Newgate are saying all sorts of things. The police are here at the picket line but it's carnage. They're looking for you.'

I fell silent.

'Are you still there? Nina, are you okay?'

'I've done a terrible thing,' I said.

'No, you haven't. *I've* done a terrible thing. I feel so ashamed. I was just protecting myself, being selfish. But I really regret it now.'

'I don't know why I did it,' I said.

She hesitated. 'What do you mean? You didn't do anything. It was me.'

I was silent.

'Nina! Are you talking about Nikolaus?'

The crowds in the background grew louder. *Pay us more! Pay us more! The UK's nurses deserve much more!*

I could hear sirens, too.

'I don't blame you, okay? Just get on with your life. I'm not holding grudges,' I said.

I hung up, clambering onto my bed. The blood rushed;

the sound of it thrashed inside my ears. Outside my window, the sirens were closing in. As I glanced up, the flicker of blue lights cut into the darkness. They shimmered across the walls like fractions of moonlight glinting upon the sea, like something predetermined.

I rose from my bed, easing myself into my coat. Whatever happened to me now didn't matter. I had to save Nikolaus.

I walked to the front door, standing there, steadying my breathing.

*I am kind and loving to myself. I am conscious of how I feel. I am ready to face up to what I did, no matter how difficult it is.*

I glanced down at my phone and sent Mercedes a text:

*You were always like a sister to me. Never forget how much I value our friendship. xx*

I heard footsteps outside, climbing up the stairs. Moments later, a heavy bang of fists on the door.

I walked towards it, calmly turning the handle.

Barry's face appeared long and drawn, but his eyes were sharp and focused. He stood with two other police officers, one man, the other a woman. I saw from their quiet expressions of resolution that this was the moment they'd all been working for.

'Nina Dabral, I am arresting you on suspicion of the murder of Leroy Gibson, unlawful disposal of a body, and perverting the course of justice by denying, when questioned by the police, that you knew the whereabouts of a missing person. You do not have to say anything, but it may harm your defence if you do not mention when questioned something which you later rely on in court. Anything you do say—'

'Just get it over with.' I held up my wrists. My body was hunched and felt so much smaller.

We walked down the stairs, Barry trotting in front, the other police officers following close.

'Can you make sure you lock up,' I called.

'No problem,' said the male officer. 'I know what it's like. So many burglaries in town.'

Outside, the sky was dark. I was swiftly ushered into a waiting police car. The air inside was stale, smelling of coffee, old Chinese takeaway cartons. But to me it offered relief. No blood or death. No smell of Newgate.

Balraj was on the pavement, observing the commotion. He caught my eye and frantically waved his hands. He shouted, 'What has happened, are you alright?' He grabbed the wheels of his wheelchair and thrust himself forward. 'Nina! Talk to me! This is a mistake, no?'

I stared down at my handcuffs as he banged his fists on the window. 'Do you need help? Are you in trouble? Can I do something? Speak to me, Nina!'

The officer beside me remained silent. The female officer in the passenger seat in front wound down the window. She urged Balraj to step away from the vehicle, to please keep at a safe distance. Sheela came running out, wheeling him back. She glanced over, her eyes narrowing at the police car.

Barry turned from the driver's seat. 'Do you understand what's happening?'

I nodded.

He sighed. 'This is a terrible situation. Not one I expected for you.' He turned back, staring out of the windscreen.

'Where's Nikolaus?' I said.

'We've questioned him. He's told us enough to implicate you in Leroy's murder.'

The other officer in front turned. I noticed her eyes, green and piercing. 'It's important you cooperate,' she said. 'The more you do, the easier it will be.'

'The press are circling,' said Barry, thumbing something onto his phone. 'It's going to come out sooner or later.' He glanced up. 'So you may as well know . . .'

'Know what?' I asked.

He was quiet for a while. 'Leroy Sanchez was an undercover policeman.' He swallowed hard, his voice breaking. 'Not just a good one, a great one.'

'What?' I struggled to breathe, my heart pounding. I felt sick.

'He was on a job, undercover. Infiltrating SK. He'd managed to find out vital information about a rival gang, but it seems he paid a terrible price. He could only play a character for so long. Of course, we've arrested suspects for his shooting. But you and I both know that's not what killed him . . .'

I dropped my head, my eyes filling as everything rushed towards me. Balraj, his stabbing seen from the bus. Dev, Farah, Mercedes, that moment I stabbed Leroy, an innocent and good man, in the stomach.

I watched a tear fall into my lap, the blot spreading like a flower in bloom. I'd got it all wrong. How ignorant and stupid could I be? I was going away for a very long time and I deserved it.

'I didn't know,' I whispered. 'You have to believe me when I say that.'

But my voice no longer felt like it was mine. Nothing I could say would ever bring Leroy back. I was distant, floating, somewhere outside myself. Observing the action from a point outside time.

From the corner of my eye, I saw Balraj wheeling his chair, the back of it pressed against the shutters of the Samosa Hut. He was talking to Farah, who stood next to Sheela to better listen. Farah was furiously scribbling notes, her hand moving swiftly over the paper, barely stopping.

'We'll do our best to manage it, but unfortunately, we can't gag journalists,' said Barry. 'Believe me, I'd love to.' The engine rumbled.

'And then what happens?' I asked, trying to prepare myself.

The female officer turned her head.

'Do you know a good lawyer?' she asked.

Barry turned the steering wheel, pulling away from the kerb.

'Only, I think you'd better get one.'

# TWO YEARS LATER

# 40

*Wednesday 25th December 2024*

*Dear Mum and Dad,*

*Rosewood Prison is privately run by an American tobacco firm. Inside, the walls are the colour of depression; hope is as far away as the sunlight of freedom. I didn't consider myself to be an evil person when I was growing up, but now, just look what happened.*

*I was sentenced to seven years for killing Leroy, a good man, a police officer. They say he was likely to have survived his shooting had I not snapped and stabbed him. Seven years for denying a man his life, the dignity of a proper burial, perverting the course of justice when the official search was underway . . .*

*The evidence they'd gathered to build a case was strong. There was no way I could defend it. Leroy's SIM. My frantic voice on the call to emergency services. Inconsistent details of my whereabouts when questioned by the police. My car spotted in the area close to the crematorium. It's almost laughable how badly organised it was. To top it off, Stefan did a runner. He's still not been found.*

*But they don't train you on how to commit murder when you're a nurse. I'm grateful Nikolaus got off more lightly with five years. When I'm out, we'll marry. That's something to live for.*

*But that's not why I'm writing.*

*I wanted to tell you that I've thought a lot about you both over the years. I used to visit the red telephone box where you left me, three times a year. I called the number a few times hoping you'd be there. Once, a stranger picked up. Public phones are for outgoing calls only, she said. That's how it's been my whole life: one-way communication.*

*I don't know if you ever followed the news after dumping me, but at the time, the police urged you both to come forward. I wasn't a newborn, they said. I had been nurtured for two weeks. I'd like to think that you had at least thought about keeping me, if only for just a few minutes.*

*The Indian lady who found me was called Kavita Dabral. She named me after her own daughter, Nina, who died at birth. Kavita died a year after she found me. Killed by a drunk driver as she walked home from work.*

*Fast-forward, life didn't exactly go to plan. But still, I can say I tried to be a good person.*

*Of course, the national papers took an interest in my origin story. They speculated whether being abandoned had affected my mental state, whether it had damaged me in some way.*

*Now, at Rosewood, I spend most of my time reading. It's something I never thought I'd do. Mills & Boon, craft magazines, sometimes articles on Labour's pledges to reform the NHS, which I'm reading with close interest.*

*In prison, they allow me use of the library and a computer. I'm allowed ten hours of surf time, weekly, with in-built site restrictions applicable. It's a privilege you must earn in here, and let's just say I've certainly earned mine.*

*One night, I googled DNA Detectives, wondering whether I should make stronger efforts to find you. I was intrigued by some of the stories that appeared:*

> I was accidentally switched at birth.
> I found my real family after forty years.
> I discovered I'm half Portuguese and Italian, with a sister I never knew I had.

*But there were other headlines, too, that made me think twice about holding on to any notion of finding you:*

> My mum's fertility doctor turned out to be my biological father.
> My real mum and dad are brother and sister.

*I've resolved to get on with my life. I'm okay not knowing who you are. I've figured you were never with me in the beginning; I should have no expectation of you being with me at the end. I'm writing you this letter on Christmas Day, more as a gift to myself. I'm rewriting the story of my life, not living somebody else's version.*

*Your daughter, Nina.*

I stare down at the woman lying on her side, skinny, pole-straight, twitching in pain, her grey prison shirt stuck to her chest, back damp with perspiration. I'm told she's been smuggling contraband in orifices not designed for storage. Small items like batteries, keys, razor blades. Even a foil sachet of tablets.

After the guards got hold of her, prising everything out, front and back, she began bleeding profusely. It's been several hours. But here, briefings are quick, no notes are kept. Everything is kept verbal, strictly off record. Their way of keeping things efficient.

Beside me, Erica rattles her keys. It's strange how working so closely with a prison guard can create a strong, familiar bond, a sense of duty and commitment.

'Make it quick, Nina. We don't want too many questions being asked.'

I glance around me. 'I'm always quick, aren't I? Been doing nights around here for long enough to know how this works.'

My hands are tired from endless work, but I pull on my gloves and fan my fingers.

Erica stands tall, jittery, a friendly, thick-limbed giant in a too-small uniform. 'Nina, I'm serious.'

'Calm down. I doubt anyone will find out,' I say. 'I'm saving you lot money by not being paid headcount.'

Erica tuts. 'I don't want a telling-off like last time.'

'They should be grateful I'm doing this at all,' I snap. I turn, opening my briefcase.

'We keep you safe in return,' she mumbles, 'along with all the *extras*.'

I glance at the woman lying on the bed, writhing in pain.

'What's your name, love?'

'Gina,' she croaks, stirring.

'I'm Nina.' But that's all I say, because too much information will only raise suspicion. I'm also acutely aware that, right now, I am a nurse, working with the worst kinds of female criminals.

'The pain is so bad; I'm gonna be sick,' says Gina, her breath fizzing behind her teeth. Her skin appears jaundiced, her eyes swollen, popping forward, almost. Her hair is frizzy and unbrushed. Her lips, dry and cracking.

I take her temperature and lean forward, noticing an angry rash blistering her skin. 'How long have you had that breakout on your face?' I ask her. 'It looks raw.'

'What breakout?' she says. 'I never even noticed it.'

Erica takes a seat in the corner, pulling out a thermos and two plastic cups from her rucksack. She pours herself tea, then kindly offers me some.

I turn to Gina once more. 'Is there anywhere else you're hurting? You must be in a lot of pain.'

But by now, Gina is so buckled up, her knees to her chest, she does not offer further explanation. When she holds up her arms, I see criss-cross cuts snaking down her wrists, ribbed as the skin healed.

'Where did you get the blades from?' I ask her gently.

'Same place.' Her mouth twists.

'Smuggled in the same way?'

She nods. 'I'm tired of working here for nothing.'

I bite my lip and stay quiet.

I rummage around my medical briefcase, full of supplies, delighting in how neat it all is. I love having my own briefcase and spend at least fifteen minutes at the end of each shift organising it for next time.

I pull out a thick dressing, a vial of antiseptic. 'I'm going to need to pull your pants down and then I'll get you cleaned up. I need to see how bad the tear is, so please remain still, if possible.'

I mop up the dried blood smeared at the back of her, squeezing the antiseptic gel on a ball of cotton wool. Gina closes her eyes, gritting her teeth.

'It burns like hell!' she cries, unable to contain it.

I peer at the slashes on her buttocks. 'I'm sorry,' I mumble. 'I'm being as gentle as I can be. I'll give you some extra-thick sanitary towels to help stop the bleeding.'

I squeeze a little Rectogesic onto a pad and dab it on the fissure. When I'm done, I replace her pants, gently easing them up.

Gina's shoulders fall. Her face relaxes. She releases a long exhale, thanking God, under her breath, that it's all over and done with.

'The good news is you don't need stitches,' I say. 'It could have been worse. I'll give you an injection for pain relief. But the cream I've just applied will help relax the muscles.'

I hear a slurp of tea and I turn, for a second expecting to see Balraj. But it's Erica, reading the front pages of a newspaper. There's an article about the results of the public inquiry into Newgate, the arrival of new leadership running the hospital. Riots in Levinstone by Reclaim England, heartwarming stories of a town, young and old, black, brown and white, uniting across cultures to tackle its community problems.

I think of Farah, her ascent to the *Guardian*, her comical expression when I told her, after several unwelcome visits, that I had no intention of allowing her to write up what happened. I'm not interested in dictating my story to her to help her sell a book. I'll write up my own story, thank you. Tell people what really happened.

I think of Mercedes, her postcard, confirming she's emigrating to Australia with Sunil.

'Where do you come from?' Gina asks after a while. 'Only, I ain't seen you before.'

'Mmm?' I'm lost in my own world.

'What you in for, I said?'

I'm sure she senses my growing discomfort. But that does not deter her. She's a cocky one, intent on prodding.

'Best not to go there,' I say. 'Here, I'm a nurse, not a criminal. That's all you need to know.'

Erica coughs to clear her throat. From the corner of my eye, I catch her smiling. But I do not further challenge her in case she withdraws my privileges. Secret phone calls to Nikolaus in Limewood Prison, five miles away. I know the value of the set-up I have here.

Around me the air grows warm and stale. I can't help but think how good it feels to be doing something important.

Gina peers at me more closely. 'Hang on . . . aren't you that nurse?'

'What nurse?'

'It *is* you, ain't it? The one they say comes in sometimes. That one done for murder.'

I rattle around my briefcase, pulling out another vial. This one is smaller and comes with an injection. I tear off the paper wrapping and hold the needle up to the light. I delight in the way the silver point glistens.

This is the part of my job I love the most, the skill, artistry, the stunning precision involved.

'Fuck off. I don't want you treating me.' Her eyes grow

wild, and she begins jerking. Behind me, Erica crosses her legs and chuckles.

'What choice do you have?' I say. 'Think they'll spend money on treating you in here? Someone with your track record of abusing your own children?'

I observe her breathing, fast and shallow. Her eyes dart about the ceiling.

'Stay calm and relax. Try to think of something else.'

But she shakes. All I can think about is how terribly inconvenient this all is, how this happens so often. I'm tired, so very tired of their predictable behaviour.

'So, what's the story with you?' I ask, attempting to distract her.

'Ended up with the wrong man, didn't I? He made me do it. I'm innocent.'

'Of course you are,' I say, clenching my jaw.

'I'm telling you, *I am.*'

I take hold of her arm, disarming her as I rub antiseptic in the crease of her elbow. 'It's like me. Everyone has got it all wrong. I tried to do the right thing, but let's just say . . . I misjudged, terribly.'

Gina stares at me strangely, her eyes narrowing. It's as if she's turning something over in her mind, and then, as reality descends, her eyes widen.

I really do love this job. They say a job should never define you, but what is there to do when there's nothing else?

I draw the needle closer as Gina screams.

'Trust me, I'm a nurse,' I say, 'it's all I ever wanted.'

# ACKNOWLEDGEMENTS

If you'd told me five years ago that I'd write a medical thriller about a nurse facing an extraordinary moral dilemma, I'd never have believed you. It's no coincidence that most medical thrillers – or rather, thrillers set in the medical world – are written by those with lived experience. When I began writing this novel, I wasn't sure whether I could ever do nursing justice. I tore my hair out and spilled blood, swearing I'd never again set a story in a hospital. But what powered me on was the motivation to write a love letter to nursing (albeit a bloody one), to acknowledge the incredible work nurses do. I was interested in exploring the split-second dilemmas nurses wrestle with daily, amid the greater challenges that come with simply doing the job: funding cuts, low wages, front-line stresses and strains. How anyone can make life-changing decisions under those circumstances was, and still is, remarkable to me.

I am enormously grateful to those who kindly shared their expertise to help me realise *The Good Patient*. To Dr Pui Yee Sophia Chan (resident doctor), Lizzy Willis (critical care outreach nurse), James Mitchell (Physio BSc), Meenaxi Patel (general manager, UCLH): thank you for helping me to understand the world of nursing and hospitals. To Debbie Peat (Nursing and Midwifery Council), thank you for our 'naughty nurses' conversation and for explaining the implications of nursing malpractice.

Special thanks to Rebecca Chalkley KC (barrister), who is a woman of considerable judicial force – and always a source of sound legal advice. Big thanks to author Chris Bridges for his much needed pedantry concerning the storage and pilfering of morphine. And finally, humble thanks to Dr Jim Down (author and consultant, UCLH), for support and guidance on questions of medical practice and procedure. If there are any mistakes or misrepresentations in this novel, those errors are entirely mine.

Thank you also to my agent, Nelle Andrew, who, despite my initial protestations, reassured me that, after writing a paedophile-hunting vigilante revenge novel, this one would be apt. To the dream team at Faber: my editor, Lochlann Binney, for their tireless efforts reading god-awful early drafts. Thank you for pushing me to finally stick in the knife, and for those tender reminders that, for a crime writer, there can be no finer outcome. I am indebted to Josephine Salverda for project-managing the almost maddening process of copy-editing precise medical details with such editorial calm and composure. And finally, thank you to Louisa Joyner, Hannah Turner and Phoebe Williams, who championed this book from the start.